Reflections on Community Psychiatric Nursing

Reflections on Community Psychiatric Nursing provides a broad range of insights into many aspects of the Community Psychiatric Nurse's (CPN's) work. Tony Gillam, writing in a fresh and accessible style, explores questions such as

- professional identity
- the community and the role of the nurse
- teaching, assessment and clinical supervision
- good practice and the concept of risk
- mental health promotion
- user involvement
- treatment, from medication to psychosocial interventions.

Written by a practising CPN, this is a lively and easy-to-read introduction to the key debates in community mental health. It will be essential reading for students and those undertaking further training as CPNs. Practising nurses and other professionals will find it helpful in developing their own reflective practice as well as offering a useful overview of an increasingly important area of nursing.

Tony Gillam is a CPN based at Kidderminster General Hospital, and is a regular contributor to nursing and mental health journals. He founded the Music Workshop Project, which won a MIND Millennium Award in 1997, and in 1998 he achieved international recognition as the UK winner of the Lilly Schizophrenia Reintegration Award.

Reflections on Community Psychiatric Nursing

Tony Gillam

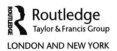

Routledge
Taylor & Francis Group

LONDON AND NEW YORK

116612723

First published 2002
by Routledge
11 New Fetter Lane, London EC4P 4EE

Simultaneously published in the USA and Canada
by Routledge
29 West 35th Street, New York, NY 10001

Reprinted 2003

Routledge is an imprint of the Taylor & Francis Group

© 2002 Tony Gillam

Typeset in Times by
M Rules
Printed and bound in Great Britain by
Biddles Ltd, Guildford and King's Lynn

British Library Cataloguing in Publication Data
A catalogue record for this book is available from the British Library

Library of Congress Cataloging in Publication Data
A catalogue record for this book has been requested

ISBN 0–415–25979–7 (pbk)
ISBN 0–415–25978–9 (hbk)

For Sue, Katie and Daniel

Contents

List of tables

Preface

Reflections on Community Psychiatric Nursing brings together a collection of previously published articles, which represent the changing trends in psychiatric nursing over the last decade. Each article is prefaced by a reflective commentary, which provides a context but also acts as an example of reflective practice. Much of the book is specifically from the perspective of a Community Psychiatric Nurse (CPN) but it is relevant to nurses from other settings and other readers with a professional or personal interest in mental health. It provides an overview of many of the major subject areas, as well as encouraging reflection and debate.

There seem to be few books available that describe contemporary psychiatric nursing and fewer, if any, which are written from the perspective of a practising CPN, rather than from that of the academic. The content of *Reflections on Community Psychiatric Nursing* provides a wide-ranging collection of discussions relating to the identity of the psychiatric nurse, concepts of community, sociological aspects of nursing and the role of the nurse compared with other mental health workers. It considers educational aspects – teaching, assessing and clinical supervision – as well as the relationship between supervision, good practice and the concept of risk. It looks at mental health promotion and user-involvement, by describing innovative interventions and projects. It explores what is 'typical' and what is 'atypical', in terms of medication and other treatments. Developments in working with families and carers are charted, as are changes in the psychiatric nurse's relationship with primary care.

In short, the scope of the book is sufficiently broad to cover many of the key areas of concern. I hope that the way the book is organised, as an anthology of articles each with its own commentary, makes for variety and readability. The commentaries provide real-life examples of reflective practice since, through these, I am reflecting on what I wrote in the original articles and why. It is a reflective, practical book rather than a book *about* reflective practice. Taken as a whole, the book provides a historical document of one psychiatric nurse's journey through a decade of change. En route, it offers much valuable information, in an easily digestible form, on a variety of themes that can then be explored further by the reader.

Acknowledgements

My thanks to all the editors of the various publications for which I have written over the past decade or so, and especially to Ian Macmillan at *Mental Health Practice* and *Nursing Standard*, Mark Radcliffe at *Nursing Times* and Catherine Jackson at *Mental Health Care*. Thanks also to all the good psychiatric nurses and mental health workers I have worked alongside, including my former team leader Sue Major and my clinical supervisor and colleague Garry Rees. To Paul Collinge for his insights into the differences between social workers and CPNs. To Russell McKie, Jasenka Horvat and Angela Fenwick for sharing their musical skill and ideas at the Birmingham Centre for Arts Therapies. To Gráinne Fadden and all the committed family therapy trainers and practitioners in the West Midlands. To Tim Salter, who I must thank for suggesting I write this book, and Matt Everett for his huge contribution to the Music Workshop Project. To the staff and volunteers of HomeStart Wyre Forest, and the staff and children of Foley Park First School. To Meredith, Patricia, Connie, Charlotte, Mark and friends at Lilly, GCI Healthcare and Cohn and Wolfe, and to Sarah Falkland and her broadcasting colleagues at BBC Radio Hereford and Worcester. Special thanks to Edwina Welham and her team at Routledge for bringing this book to fruition.

To all other family, friends, colleagues and patients whom I have not named but who have shared so much with me.

Permissions

A large part of this book has already appeared in the form of articles in various periodicals. I would like to acknowledge and thank the following for kind permission to re-use this material in book form.

The following articles appeared originally in *Nursing Times*: 'Teaching and learning in lay-bys' in the *Nursing Times Learning Curve* supplement (3 September 1997, Vol. 1, No. 7); 'Taking a humanistic approach to assessment' in the *Nursing Times Learning Curve* supplement (3 December 1997, Vol. 1, No. 10); 'Clinical supervision' as a 'clinical view' column (9 September 1998, Vol. 94, No. 36); 'Discontinuation syndrome', also as a 'clinical view' column (10 March 1999, Vol. 95, No. 10); 'Song sung blue', which originally appeared alongside 'Second that emotion' (6 October 1999, Vol. 95, No. 40); 'Sounds good' (9 October 1996, Vol. 94, No. 41); and 'Too close for comfort?' (30 September 1998, Vol. 94, No. 39).

The following articles appeared originally in *Nursing Standard*: 'Psychiatric nursing in the community' (25 October 1989, Vol. 4, No. 5); 'Unemployment links with mental health' (12 May 1993, Vol. 7, No. 34); 'Get the bucket and mop, nurse' (26 May 1993, Vol. 7, No. 36); 'The role of community mental health workers' (18 May 1994, Vol. 8, No. 34); 'Risk-taking: a nurse's duty' (19 June 1991, Vol. 5, No. 39); 'What's it worth?' (8 February 1995, Vol. 9, No. 20); 'Representational systems in counselling' (24 November 1993, Vol. 8, No. 10); 'CPN'd of the line?' (26 January 1994, Vol. 8, No. 18); and 'Family therapy – exploring the role of the CPN' (3 June 1996, Vol. 10, No. 24).

'Working with HomeStart' appeared originally in *Mental Health Practice* (March 2000, Vol. 3, No. 6).

'Diary of a Community Psychiatric Nurse' was first published by *The Guardian* (Wednesday 10 March 1999).

'"Community" and "neighbourhood" – how concepts shape the provision of care' was published originally in the *Community Psychiatric Nurses Journal* (August 1991, Vol. 11, No. 4, 12–16).

'Atypical antipsychotics – a psychiatric nurse's perspective' appeared originally in a key paper review in *Progress in Neurology and Psychiatry* (Jan./Feb. 2000, Vol. 4, No. 1). A version of 'The case for using family interventions in the management of schizophrenia' is currently in press and is due to appear in *Progress in Neurology and Psychiatry*.

'Creative arts as therapy' was published originally in *Nursing* (27 September –10 October 1990, Vol. 4, No. 1).

The following articles appeared originally in *Mental Health Care*: 'Putting innovation on the map' as 'Into the breach' (June 2000, Vol. 3, No. 10) and one of the 'Two case studies of psychoeducational family interventions' as 'Listening to what Simon says' (March 2001, Vol. 1, No. 7).

'Managing depression in primary care' was published originally in *The Journal of Primary Care Mental Health* (2000, Vol. 4, No. 1).

1 Who was that masked man?

The identity of the Community Psychiatric Nurse

Reflection

By the late 1980s I was living in an old hospital house in the grounds of a Victorian asylum – Powick Hospital in Worcester. I was working on nights as a newly qualified staff nurse at the city's modern Newtown Hospital but the only accommodation my wife and I had been offered by my new employer was one of a row of unfurnished houses with no heating and a leaking roof. A few years later it was demolished, along with Powick Hospital itself.

In that first cold winter in Worcester, I had come across an article in the *Nursing Standard* on 'How to write a book review'. The book reviews editor, Phyllis Holbrook, was – it seemed to me – trying to encourage readers to become book reviewers, so I tried my luck and began to have the first of many reviews published. Spurred on by this, I decided to try writing an article and, searching for ideas, came across something I had written in my final year as a student nurse.

While on student placement with the Community Psychiatric Nurses in Telford I had been asked to 'give a little talk' on an aspect of community psychiatric nursing. I read it through and it looked passable, so I typed it up on an ancient manual typewriter that my father-in-law had given me, and sent it off to *Nursing Standard*. By the time it was published (in October 1989) we had moved house and had a baby, and I had escaped from night duty by changing health authorities once again, this time taking a job as a staff nurse in an acute psychiatric day hospital in Kidderminster.

I felt I had been rehabilitated, moving from nights onto days, and from in-patient to day-patient services. There was a record in the charts at the time by Soul II Soul called *Back to Life*. The opening lines were, 'Back to life, back to reality . . .' I was delighted to be able to work in therapeutic groups and to do one-to-one counselling with day patients who lived in the community. After some time in day care, I had the opportunity of being completely rehabilitated into the community. I took the leap that several of those day patients were fearing and left the relative security of the day hospital team for the breathtaking freedom of becoming a Community Psychiatric Nurse (CPN) in my own right. It felt like an enormous privilege to have so much autonomy and so much responsibility.

Over the intervening years I have glanced at that first article from time to time and have felt a little embarrassed. Was it not a bit presumptuous of me to suggest how CPNs should work when, at the time of writing, I was not even a CPN? Was I not romanticising the job of the CPN, by making a CPN out to be some kind of Lone Ranger or a Philip Marlowe-style private investigator?

A while ago, re-reading it by way of preparation for this book, I decided I should stand by this first article. After all, it was written from the point of view of a student nurse and from the perspective of one who had spent more time working in hospital than working in the community. I think these are important viewpoints from which to comment upon what CPNs do and the article touches on some key concerns for CPNs then and now.

The blossoming of private-finance initiatives and public–private collaboration has meant that the centralisation of health services has continued despite the decentralising impulse of community care. It remains to be seen if any kind of National Service Framework can force providers to balance 'economies of scale' with the wishes of people to have a 'local' service. Over the past decade we have seen a resurgence in the debate about compulsory treatment in the community, so the concept of CPNs as 'community custodians', however distasteful, is relevant. The tension between autonomy and teamwork is as alive as ever, no less so with the emergence of community mental health teams. Plenty of CPNs continue to lead remarkably autonomous professional lives, some with a 'take-it-or-leave-it' attitude to clinical supervision and accountability. The idea of assertive leadership that promotes autonomy and teamwork seems even more imperative now that I am a practising CPN than it did when I looked on, admiringly, from the vantage point of the hospital-trained student nurse.

Psychiatric nursing in the community – the Lone Ranger and the multi-disciplinary team

In the traditional psychiatric institution the services are centralised: all roads lead to hospital, so to speak. A patient is identified in the community, his or her illness becomes acute and the patient is admitted to the hospital where all the resources are concentrated in one place.

According to the more modern, patient-centred approach, services should be decentralised and, to avoid institutionalising patients, the services should come to the people. Those who see psychiatry as a means of social control might see this as a shift in the psychiatric nurse's role from custodian/ warden to vigilante. The community nurse goes out in search of the problem people, in an attempt to 'clean up the city'. The CPN seeks to eradicate psychiatric problems, to get to the root of the problem and thus to purge the community.

Whether or not we subscribe to this anti-psychiatry view of community nursing it cannot be denied that a major source of satisfaction for the CPN is going out there and doing the job on his or her own. The CPNs are lone rangers, their own boss, and any successes are entirely to their personal credit.

CPNs seem to take pride in the fact that they dispense with their colleagues' opinions, they are freethinkers, private investigators trying to get a lead to solve the mystery of mental illness, shunning interference from other agencies.

The difficulty with this attitude is that it is hard to reconcile it with the 'team approach'. The concept of working as a member of a multi-disciplinary team, pooling skills and resources, has become central to modern hospital nursing. It has many advantages for both patients and staff. From the staff point of view it means shared responsibility and shared accountability, and helps to avoid the disillusionment and exhaustion that contribute to burnout. From the patient's viewpoint there is the benefit of specialised help from a number of different perspectives. A second opinion is not something that has to be sought but something offered automatically.

Perhaps an ideal combination, then, would be a fusion of the independent worker approach with the team approach. This would mean a commitment on the part of the CPN to build up group cohesion with his colleagues.

Regular and frequent meetings are one way of ensuring continuity of care but also improve communication and, at best, should reassure nurses of the mutual support they can offer one another. It should not be thought of as a weakness to admit difficulties and to seek practical help and moral support. On the contrary, to be able to discuss freely in this way is a hallmark of professionalism.

Meetings should be equally concerned with sorting out business and building group cohesion. Important as it is, making time for meetings will not on its own guarantee group cohesion or ensure that CPNs work as a team. It is essential that the team has firm leadership to keep it together.

The question of leadership is not clear cut in community nursing. In a hospital ward the structured hierarchy means that everyone knows where they stand. But if it is desirable for each member of the team to have an equal say, for one opinion to be as valid as any other, then the most senior cannot afford to pull rank and the most junior cannot afford to abdicate their share of responsibility.

What is called for is a flattening of the hierarchy. There is a boss, but not a bossy boss, there are junior nurses but they are not mere errand-runners, tea-makers, yes men or scapegoats. A flattened hierarchy seems the ideal framework for a team approach, where everyone listens to and respects everybody else. Although people are accountable for their own actions, the team still needs to be overseen and directed if it is not to disintegrate at times.

The senior nurse's responsibility is to ensure that rifts are healed, communication lines are kept open, ideas are exchanged, feelings expressed, and grievances aired freely and constructively. As team leaders, it is their job to encourage people to work together and look after one another.

Bearing in mind that, from what has already been discussed, CPNs are notorious for going their own way, it will be clear that at times this 'encouragement' will need to be quite forceful. They may need to be chased and cajoled into making time for meetings. Once captured, CPNs may need to be probed and prompted to discuss things and, in sharing difficulties, protected against feeling that they are admitting failure and defeat. If nurses and services are not to break down and burn out then these solitary, pioneering creatures somehow need their independence respected and their professionalism shared.

2   No such thing as society

Sociological aspects of community psychiatric nursing

Reflection

Any discussion about what job title best describes the CPN these days seems to centre on whether we are Community *Psychiatric* Nurses or Community *Mental Health* Nurses. Do we want to continue to be associated with psychiatry, and would it not be better if we focused on mental health rather than mental illness? This is a debate taken up by Liam Clarke in his book *Challenging Ideas in Psychiatric Nursing*. Clarke describes the recommendation that all psychiatric nurses should be awarded the title 'mental health nurse' as 'quite astonishing for whatever chance one might have of defining mental illness, defining mental health . . . would be a formidable task indeed' (Clarke 1999: 9). He suggests that, given that all three terms ('community', 'psychiatric' and 'nurse') are 'problematic', any analysis of community psychiatric nursing must deal with the meanings to which these words give rise.

When I first became a CPN I was less concerned about the 'P' and the 'N' and more interested in the 'C'. I was curious about the community I was serving. Where was it? What was it? The first of these questions might be solved with a good street map, but the second was more philosophical. I commuted each day to work and, at the end of the afternoon, would return to my own 'community' – an area called St John's in Worcester. Except, I was not sure if this really was *my community*. I lived there, I was registered with a doctor there, I used the local post office and bakery, but I did not know my neighbours, I knew nothing of the history of the area and was unsure whether I would stay there for the rest of my life.

In TV soaps, like *EastEnders* and *Coronation Street*, everybody seems to use the same pub, the same café. I did not. I discovered one pub in St John's where I felt very welcome. This was the Brunswick Arms, where they had folk music every Sunday night. I think I felt so comfortable there, not because it was a stone's throw from my house and not because it was in my part of town, but because other musicians went there. I had found my community. A community of musicians, many of whom did not live in the neighbourhood at all.

In the article, '"Community" and "neighbourhood"', I not only question these concepts but explore different ways of working for community nurses. At that time, our CPN team had a referral system that allowed each CPN to take on those referrals they found interesting. There was a weekly meeting in which all the referrals that had been received (probably between two and five) would be discussed. CPNs would then make bids for them, taking into account how busy they were, any annual leave coming up, any special interests in either the patients' conditions or suggested approaches to dealing with these.

A number of things happened that changed this. One was a growing reluctance among some of the team members to take on referrals, forcing others to take them by default. This illustrates the potential for the abuse of autonomy in community psychiatric nursing. The second change was the introduction of GP-attachment, which meant that patients started to be allocated, not in terms of special interest, particular skills or caseload capacity, but according to whether the referral came from the practice to which you were attached. Inevitably, some practices refer more often than others, which creates inequalities within teams. Thirdly, when I reflect back to our old referral meetings, I realise that there were actually fewer referrals coming into the team in those days. This meant that we had the luxury (if that is what it was) of carefully considering the appropriateness of a handful of referrals each week and how best to allocate them. Finally, there was something introduced called 'Patient's Charter Standards', which set similar standards for community nurses of all kinds, CPNs, district nurses and midwives, lumping us all together in a frenzy to meet the needs of 'urgent' and 'non-urgent' referrals. It seems to me that there is a difference between an emergency for a midwife and an emergency for a CPN but this was not taken into account. Thus, our calm, collected and delightfully civilised way of dealing with people in possible need of the skills of a CPN was replaced with the feast or famine that is the lot of a GP-attached CPN. The trend towards Community Mental Health Teams may well mean a move back to a more rational way of allocating referrals but it would seem that the community of people deemed to be in need of a CPN continues to grow.

'Community' and 'neighbourhood' – how concepts shape the provision of care

Phrases such as 'community care' and 'neighbourhood watch' have entered so much into common parlance in recent years that we have perhaps lost sight of the values implied. It has been said that the term 'community' has been used 'with an abandon reminiscent of poetic licence' (Wirth 1979). The words 'community' and 'neighbourhood' have an almost quaint connotation. They imply a return to a simpler way of life, where people cared for each other, far from the self-centred hustle and bustle of modern life. Dennis protests, however, that 'the usefulness of the idea of the neighbourhood community is not commensurate with the kind of popularity . . . it enjoys' (Dennis 1968). Dennis suggests that the words' resurgence in the latter part of this century has not been accompanied by a resurgence in their concomitant values. This may constitute a form of what Piaget called 'magical thinking' on the part of planners and politicians, whereby simply using the words brings about a change in attitude (Piaget 1929). The same principle applies to the preference for the phrase 'mental health' over 'mental illness' – the aim is to shift the emphasis, to re-frame in a positive light. In this case, it could be that 'mental health workers', such as CPNs, are equally guilty of magical thinking – wishing we dealt in mental health, rather than with mental illness.

As CPNs we need to ask, 'Where is the community in which we work?' or, indeed, 'What is the community?' It is here that sociology can help us. Sociology has no shortage of definitions of the term. 'At the minimum [community] . . . refers to a collection of people in a geographical area' (Abercrombie *et al.* 1988). Many definitions extend to include concepts such as a sense of belonging and of self-containment. For example, MacIver and Page (1961) write that 'the bases of community are *locality* and *community sentiment*', whereas nowadays we find

> people occupying specific local areas which lack the social coherence necessary to give them a community character. For example, the residents of a ward or district of a large city may lack sufficient contacts or common interests to instil conscious identification with the area. Such a 'neighbourhood' is not a community because it does not possess a feeling of belonging together. . . . There must be the common living with its *awareness* of sharing a way of life as well as the common earth.
>
> (MacIver and Page 1961)

This insistence on identification and belongingness seems to have its origins in earlier concepts of *Gemeinschaft* and *Gesellschaft* (Toennies 1955). Toennies suggested that traditional/rural societies had a sense of community (Gemeinschaft), whereas modern/urban society (Gesellschaft) tended to be more individualistic and impersonal. Relationships in Gemeinschaft were seen as close, supportive and affective, whereas in Gesellschaft relationships were distanced and merely contractual. Gemeinschaft, then, implies collective identity and solidarity: 'it is the lasting and genuine form of living together', wrote Toennies, 'in contrast to Gemeinschaft, Gesellschaft is transitory and superficial' (Toennies 1955).

Few CPNs, I suggest, would describe the communities they serve as Gemeinschaften in Toennies' sense. Some CPNs would concede that their community at least fits the minimal definition of a 'collection of people in a geographical area' (Abercrombie *et al.* 1988). I recently attended an event called a 'Community Lunch'. A district nurse discovered I was a CPN and asked, making polite conversation, if this was my 'patch'. I bemused her by trying to explain that our team had shunned the 'patch' system and, instead, allocated referrals on the basis of 'I feel I could work with this client'. By this means, the phrase 'this case is right up my street' becomes figurative rather than literal. The result of this trend, however, is that many CPNs cannot even claim to fulfil the minimum definition of community. Perhaps we may work in 'neighbourhoods', in MacIver and Page's sense – areas lacking an 'awareness of sharing a way of life'.

If community is more than a myth, it soon becomes clear that we need more sophisticated definitions. If these cannot save the concept, the term is redundant in our job title.

Louis Wirth (1979) defined community as a 'constellation of institutions. These include not merely . . . schools, churches [etc.] . . . but also such phenomena as families, . . . clubs . . . and recreation centres'. This begins to sound like something with which a CPN could work – engaging the family in the client's treatment, helping the client make contact with local drop-in centres. Familiar territory. Better still, Wirth offers an alternative view of community in what he calls a 'social-psychological approach'. This sees community as 'a constellation of types of personalities'. He suggests the institutions mentioned above need to be supplemented by 'the more subjective material to be obtained only through personal contact with . . . human beings'. This subjective material might be the variable that dooms more simplistic conceptions to failure. Wirth seems to be saying that culture is at least as important as human geography.

Geography may, in fact, have little to do with community. Webber (1979) suggested that 'communities comprise people with common interests who communicate with each other'. In this 'non-place', what he calls 'physical propinquity' has nothing to do with 'a sense of belonging'.

In order to test out the practical implications of these definitions for community nursing, I would like to consider them in the light of a document called *Neighbourhood Nursing – A Focus for Care* (Cumberlege *et al.* 1986). In this report, the Community Nursing Review Team proposed a 'new idea': 'Each district health authority should identify within its boundaries neighbourhoods for the purpose of planning, organising and providing nursing and related primary care services'. Neighbourhood is defined here as consisting of a population of between 10,000 and 25,000, these being the smallest and largest numbers that constitute 'a viable neighbourhood for the purposes proposed'. These are no Gemeinschaften but may fit MacIver and Page's definition of neighbourhood.

What interests us here is the ideological significance of re-naming community nursing as neighbourhood nursing. Was it born of a disillusionment with the idea of community? Not at all. *Neighbourhood Nursing* quotes approvingly from the National Council for Voluntary Organisations: 'Providing effective care and health advice means recognising that individuals are part of their communities'. They recommend that community nurses gain an understanding of community networks in order to utilise local self-help groups.

Again, we find ourselves idealising community. A CPN may know of a MIND drop-in centre round the corner from his anxious client's house but, if the client sees himself as not belonging to a community of mentally ill people (in Webber's sense of community), this may not be at all appropriate. The drop-in may comprise people from several different neighbourhoods, while the anxious client – although living in the same neighbourhood as the centre – belongs to a different community. In its effort to respond to 'local need', *Neighbourhood Nursing* inadvertently makes us blind to individual need, on one level, and (on another) to broader societal forces.

It is naive to believe that a collection of houses must form a meaningful social unit. Dennis (1968) explores the origins of our love affair with the idea and traces it to those nineteenth-century commentators who argued it was convenient to fragment the masses into 'localities'. The implication is that the over-concentration of working-class people in cities posed a real threat of an uprising. Thus, it suited the ruling class, politically and psychologically, to encourage an identification with one's own local community. The alternative might be to allow working-class people in one locality to show solidarity with the rest of the working class, regionally, nationally and internationally. Described in this way, community is an antidote to revolution – or perhaps to any kind of genuine social change:

> The locality-community idea implies fixing one's eyes on the part local factors play in the aetiology of social and personal problems, and it pre-sumes that these problems can be dealt with by . . . applying psychotherapeutic measures to persons who work and live in the problem locality. This is obviously not a very threatening thing to do . . . it does not present a challenge to any fundamental institutions or established social beliefs. It does not appear to involve the examination of the con-tribution of more general social-structural and cultural factors.
>
> (Dennis 1968)

Is the *community* psychiatric nurse standing in the way of revolution? By virtue of our job title alone, do we perpetuate a myth that inhibits social change? If those of us who work within the 'patch' system imagine for one moment that our client group must be homogenous, then we could certainly be held guilty of this – and of the crassest form of stereotyping. Again, if we follow the logic of *Neighbourhood Nursing* by referring clients to the nearest, rather than the most appropriate, drop-in centre, we might as well join Margaret Thatcher in her contention that there is no such thing as society.

Of course, economics enters into community nursing. The 'patch' system saves on travelling expenses (even if the CPN with a special interest in alco-hol abuse works on the other side of town from your alcoholic client for whom you have no great empathy). The Health Visitors' Association has been particularly critical of un-rationalised caseload management, as were Mrs Cumberlege's team:

> Particularly in urban areas, doctors' lists can include patients living many miles apart, scattered across large towns or areas of cities and straddling

health authority borders. In extreme cases . . . 15 or 20 general practitioners may be caring for as few as 50 households in one tower block with the result that many different health visitors will be calling at the same location.

(Cumberlege *et al.* 1986)

Presumably, one health visitor is as good as another and one health visitor is quite enough for one tower block. Fifty households, however, may have very varied needs. Unless health visitors are considerably more talented than CPNs it seems unlikely that one health visitor would have all the skills and resources to meet that variety of needs. I visit several households in a tower block which is also visited by most of my CPN colleagues at one time or another. I would argue that the clients living there get the CPN they need. By the same token I would uphold those clients' right to choose the GP who suits their needs, in contrast to *Neighbourhood Nursing* which 'hopes' that the zoning of GP practices will spread.

Community nursing is not just about economics. It is about choice. There is a world of difference between 'neighbourhood' and 'zone'. People *belong* to neighbourhoods but they are *put* in zones, and have little choice over which zone they are zoned into. Under the National Health Service and Community Care Act 1990, GPs have the choice of which zone to care for. Already there is the case of three doctors in Carlisle deciding to exclude two council estates from their general practice because they believed the residents to be 'the sort that tend not to attend for cervical smears and immunisation' and thus likely to prevent them from reaching screening targets and bonus payments (Cobb 1990: 9). Neighbourhoods with a high concentration of schizophrenia sufferers might equally be considered undesirable zones.

Ultimately, organising care for the mentally ill in terms of community, neighbourhood or zone may be less helpful than organising it in terms of individual choice. By this, I mean choice for the users of the NHS, not the providers. In an essay entitled 'Community Care', Sue Townsend wrote:

I have yet to find the community that is prepared to help and care for the recovering mentally ill. There will always be saintly individuals and voluntary groups who do wonderful unrecognised work with the mentally ill, but the larger community? Forget it. They get up petitions *against* hostels. They do *not* care. The ex-patients, the unofficial street entertainers . . . need protecting *against* the community.

(Townsend 1989)

Perhaps the mentally ill need rescue at two levels: not so much from the *people* who make up a locality as from the *idea* of the neighbourhood community. They need rescuing from the ideology that 'presumes these problems can be dealt with without challenging any fundamental institutions or established social beliefs' (Dennis 1968). They need rescuing from 'neighbourhood nurses' who focus on local needs before individual needs; from health visitors who want patients zoned. They need rescuing from GPs who refuse, out of hand, to care for whole council estates.

If community psychiatric nursing is to serve the interests of the mentally ill, we need to be wary of making assumptions about individuals based on locality. We need to maintain choices for the mentally ill despite economic and political constraints. Above all, we need to recognise the extent to which 'community' is a myth and to consider that the interests served by this myth are unlikely to be the interests of the mentally ill.

Reflection

When the mental health editor of *Nursing Standard* asked me to write a feature about the problems that 'spiralling unemployment' was causing in 1993, I had no shortage of material on which to draw. So many of my patients were struggling to find employment, whether they were school leavers or middle-aged victims of recession made redundant. It felt like history repeating itself, as I reflected back to my own days of signing on ten years earlier.

Looking back with yet another decade's hindsight, I am struck by the changes that have taken place. At the time of writing this reflection, employment is high in the UK, to the point where there is a recruitment crisis in the public sector. Graduates – even arts graduates like my ne'er-do-well companions and I – are much less likely to resort to careers in teaching, let alone nursing these days. Higher education does indeed seem to correlate with more than adequate employment prospects, which is just as well considering today's students approach their degrees in a workmanlike fashion, without grants and with loans.

I cannot imagine what it is like to be a full-time undergraduate in this climate. Students used to have the choice of living frugally on benefits between terms or finding a job. Now the benefits have stopped but the promise of graduate employment is there to pay off the loans. No one is unemployed any more, everyone is a 'jobseeker'. I have patients – women in their fifties – who used to be called housewives but who are now encouraged to overcome their depression and anxiety to work a few hours a week for part of their benefits. Perhaps this is an acknowledgement of the link between work and mental health but I belong to an age, not so far back in time, when students might be poor but eventually started their working lives debt-free and when people of a certain age were allowed not to have a job if that made more sense.

Unemployment links with mental health

In the early 1980s it was not unusual for university graduates to experience several months of unemployment after completing a degree. This did not please my brother who felt he had paid enough in taxes to finance four years of higher education and was dismayed to see that instead of finding highly taxable graduate employment, I promptly signed on. So did many of my friends, until we eventually found work as teachers, social workers, even as psychiatric nurses. There was a certain irony in the fact that our escape from unemployment was to work for the welfare state, which existed partly to support those less able to escape.

Among the recommended texts for budding Registered Mental Nurses (RMNs) was *Sociology for Nurses*, which stated in 1982: 'One person in ten is unemployed in Britain and there are signs that this may result in increased illness and death' (Chapman 1982: 75). Those of us versed in pop music already knew this statistic, thanks to the band UB40's 1982 hit, *One in Ten*. The group named themselves after the card issued to people claiming unemployment benefit. The album sleeve boasted a twelve-inch replica of this all too familiar item. It was disturbing when, a decade later, *One in Ten* was re-issued, finding relevance to a new generation.

Another recommended text, *A Short Textbook of Psychiatry*, boldly stated: 'Loss of work constitutes a stress and may tax the adaptive capacity of the person to the maximum, particularly if it means marked loss of financial status, marked loss of prestige, or creates additional problems with the family' (Rees 1982: 66).

In the days before the NHS 'reforms', nursing offered an enviable degree of job security. Student nurses were offered staff nurse posts as a matter of course. Part of this security came from the anomaly that the NHS was not subject to market forces. But part of it, particularly for psychiatric nurses, was based on the macabre twist that illness, and especially mental illness, often seems to be the only growth industry during a recession. Not only did nurses service the casualties of socio-economic disaster, they also depended on them for their own job security. Hence, my father's cheery assertion: 'They will always want nurses'. True, no doubt, but will 'they' always be willing to pay for highly qualified, well-trained nurses, or would a care assistant do?

All I know is that newly qualified nurses no longer find work without delay. And, for the first time, the word 'redundancy' describes something happening to nursing staff instead of a life event exclusive to some patients. My textbook (Rees 1982) spoke dispassionately of the 'psychological sequelae to the event of unemployment'. Re-reading it now, it appears bizarre that the symptoms can be recounted as though they are the surprising result of a rare disease.

As a CPN working in a town devastated by unemployment, the facts of my caseload are unsurprising. Out of more than 30 clients, 75 per cent are unemployed. It could be argued that unemployment is an effect of some of these people's illnesses, rather than a precipitating factor. But for many, it seems to be the other way around – their mental health problems have arisen *since* being made redundant. This does not mean that unemployment causes mental illness. Were the argument so simplistic, it would follow that finding work cures mental illness.

Yet, on one level, this has the ring of truth. One of my clients seemed to be experiencing an abnormal grief reaction after the death of a relative and was judged to be a suicide risk. My initial assessment was that he would need a prolonged period of counselling to work through difficulties in his family and problems with his sexual identity. All this was unnecessary, however, because the client announced a few visits later that he had been offered a job he had always wanted. Naturally, I was sceptical that everything had suddenly been set to right and offered a few more sessions, anticipating that the euphoria would subside and the original problems re-emerge. However, it became clear that finding a job had transformed the way he felt about his bereavement, his family and himself.

This experience taught me that when clients say, 'I'd be all right if I could just find a job', they may be right. I would be failing in my job if I did not challenge this apparently concrete, psychologically unsophisticated rationalisation. Nevertheless, employment is a concrete, psychologically unsophisticated matter for many people. Marxists may argue that employment is an alienating experience, exhausting people's energies while denying them control over their labour and its products. But a common theme that has arisen in a therapeutic group I run for men has been that the only thing more alienating than work is the lack of it.

The group members all have mental health problems, predominantly anxiety and depression. Their unemployment rate has remained 100 per cent over a twelve-month period. Depressive feelings of worthlessness run deep among them and anxiety over social situations worsens as opportunities to work diminish. Their marriages become increasingly strained, as men lose their self-concept as the main provider and feel guilty or jealous as their wives continue to work. Loss of confidence and lack of practice may result in a loss of skills, which, in turn, leads to a greater loss of self-esteem. I hear about the 'psychological sequelae of unemployment' every week in the group.

Group members refer to being made redundant as 'the time when I was finished'. This is used not only as an adjective but also as an intransitive verb, so that 'to finish' means 'to make redundant'. It is a sure sign of powerlessness when verbs that most of us use transitively ('I'll finish work at 5 p.m.') are used intransitively ('They finished me just before Christmas').

A new development is that CPNs are now receiving referrals from the Jobcentre or, to be precise, the Disability Employment Advisor. There was a time when psychiatrists would refer a patient to the then Disability Resettlement Officer (DRO). It is no longer a case of resettling people into the world of work they left temporarily during their mental illness. The DRO's change of title implies that the working world is an unsettled and unsettling place where advice on employment is no guarantee of finding a job.

Referrals from the advisors often provide an opportunity for early intervention in mental health problems. But the public may be alarmed to learn that people are being referred directly from the Jobcentre to psychiatric services. It is as if the state is admitting: 'We cannot find you a job, but we understand this causes you a lot of stress. Perhaps you need psychiatric help.'

In some cases, it seems the CPN's task is to make unemployment more bearable for the individual, and less of a problem for government and society. CPNs may help clients to claim unclaimed benefits, refer people to the Disability Employment Advisor or encourage them to engage in voluntary work. Voluntary work can improve a person's mental health but it must be treated with caution. As one group member justly pointed out: 'It's all right this volunteer centre co-ordinator coming to the day hospital encouraging us to do voluntary work, but *she* is getting paid, isn't she?'

There is a danger that voluntary work and government training schemes could be used as a form of community-orientated industrial therapy. Any substitute for 'real jobs' can lead to exploitation and, at the very least, detract from the real problem. An effective government policy to reduce unemployment may have been more helpful than any number of documents on *The Health of the Nation*. Now, with nurses joining the ranks of the unemployed, the health of the nation looks sicker by the day. At least society seems to be more aware of the 'one in tens'. I only hope my old textbooks were right when they said that awareness of a problem is the first step on the road to recovery.

Reflection

The article 'Get the bucket and mop, nurse' can best be described as a 'rant'. I was driving to work one day in 1993, listening to *Today* on Radio Four. I remember a couple of politicians discussing the need for pay restraint in the public sector and arguing that essentially unproductive workers could not expect to get pay rises that were in line with inflation. It seemed to me nurses were being punished for choosing a career that made nothing useful, not even money. To add insult to injury, on the other hand, politicians were arguing that the NHS had to become more businesslike, that it should not be exempt from market forces.

In the heyday of health authorities applying to be in this or that wave of Trust status, and GPs getting excited about being 'fund-holding' little business empires, there suddenly developed an unhealthy obsession with quantitative measures of what CPNs did. I remember arguing with a practice manager of a local GP surgery. She insisted that the information I had supplied to her was full of clerical errors because it looked as if I had visited the same patient three times in one day. I assured her that I had used a considerable amount of my own clinical time to enter this data on computer and I was certain, as regards that particular patient, it was accurate. 'But it can't be right!' she insisted, 'you wouldn't visit the same patient three times in one day!' I tried to explain that indeed I had, the reason being that the patient was elusive and chaotic, and was often not in at the agreed times but that he was on a depot injection which he needed that day, so I had persevered. 'We quite often visit people several times a day', I explained. 'Sometimes the people we visit don't want to see us, they forget, they go out, they pretend not to be in. We spend a lot of time chasing people, and even more recording that information in the form of statistics so that you can see how hard we work for you.'

Subsequent governments have tried hard to soften the impact of the market on public servants, to encourage the retention of nurses 'at the bedside', as politicians say, and of teachers 'at the chalk-face'. Nevertheless, while playing 'catch-up' after years of pay restraint, there has been a growing insistence on 'value for money' and professional accountability, which has drowned the helping professions in a tidal wave of initiatives and guidelines and so many 'tools' to enhance good practice that many decide the task is impossible.

Get the bucket and mop, nurse

'Who wants to be a nurse when she grows up?' asks the schoolteacher in Garrison Keillor's comic novel *Lake Wobegon Days*, when a boy vomits on the floor:

> 'Nurses help sick people in many different ways', she tells Betty as they walk to the lunchroom. 'They have many different jobs to do. Now here is one of them. The mop is in the kitchen. Be sure to use plenty of Pine-Sol.'

(Keillor 1986: 14)

The teacher might have told Betty about regulatory bodies, such as the United Kingdom Central Council for Nurses (UKCC). Nurses in the UK dutifully pay periodic registration fees for the privilege of remaining on the register. This also entitles them to receive the UKCC's exciting bulletin, *Register*, an issue of which I have before me. It contains an article on nurse prescribing (UKCC 1992: 7). From it we learn that the right to prescribe from a limited range of drugs will initially be restricted to qualified district nurses and health visitors.

Although I am not anxious to acquire prescriptive powers, I do sometimes find myself chasing around the hospital in search of a junior doctor to sign a prescription sheet for a patient in the community. The patient is often not known to the doctor. The medication that I know needs to be re-prescribed is not necessarily one the doctor is familiar with but, when I explain the dose and the frequency required, he or she always signs obligingly. There is no reason not to. The doctor bows to my long-standing acquaintance with the patient and my experience in psychiatry, which spans considerably more years than his or hers.

The article in *Register* makes no mention of psychiatric nurses. No matter. The lofty heights of prescribing powers are far from the minds of CPNs like myself. CPNs are much more concerned with no less a task than justifying their existence. In the free market NHS, business managers need proof of our productivity. They have set us to work on that most important of tasks – recording the number of visits we make.

Proof of high 'activity' rates will help sell the product to the service's purchasers, fundholding GPs. They are the ones with real power. They can acquire for patients all the mental healthcare money can buy. CPNs could have pride of place in the company. They are potentially the primary sales force of new trusts.

Nurses everywhere should be forgiven for reflecting upon the fact that they could have applied for clerical jobs if they had wanted to fill in forms all day. There is a growing sense that our role is being defined, not by other professions as has traditionally been the case, but by the forces of the market and the discipline of managerialism.

Most nurses still feel they want to provide a health service to the public. They are public servants who have often had to perform the most menial tasks in their service to people. This brings us back to the unfortunate Betty. Nurses do indeed have many different jobs to do – collecting statistics, perhaps prescribing drugs, and certainly marketing their service. But it still helps if you are handy with a mop and bucket.

Those higher-paid public servants in the government have decreed that nurses in the public sector have had it too good for too long. Shielded from the recession and, until recently, from market forces, nurses have avoided the insecurity that those in really important jobs have had to endure. As punishment, we have had disregarded the recommendations of our Pay Review Body. This will give industry the chance to pull the UK out of recession without having to pay all those unproductive people in that pesky health service. Nurses are literally paying the price for being part of the public service.

You will recall that there was once a NHS. In spite of professional rivalries, things were not too bad. Then came market forces and suddenly there was a terrible mess. Somebody has made a terrible mess. And it stinks. Pass the disinfectant.

Reflection

In 1994 it seemed conceivable that market forces, which measured health care in terms of completed episodes of in-patient care, could make CPNs obsolete. This was long before New Labour declared encouragingly that community care had failed! Could community psychiatric nursing go out of favour? It seemed absurd and yet we were being pummelled by the twin forces of GP fundholding and health authorities' quest for Trust status. This made me take stock of just how much was expected of CPNs, what made us unique and what was to become of us. Some witty sub-editor at *Nursing Standard* coined the phrase 'CPN'd of the line', but it was not all inevitable doom and gloom. The addition of the question mark at the end of the headline 'CPN'd of the line?' suggested that it might not be.

Re-visiting this article now, I recall my attempts to engage the family of the patient described though, at that time, my involvement of the family was based on a feeling that it was instinctively right, rather than influenced by the impressive body of evidence for family interventions (see Chapter 10). The other striking thing is the very broad range of client group described. This may still accurately reflect the varied workload of CPNs as a group but my impression is that, these days, CPN services are more targeted (there are CPNs for 'acute', 'recovery', 'early intervention', 'assertive outreach', 'GP liaison', etc.) so it may be harder to find individual CPNs with vastly mixed caseloads.

Working with severe and enduring mental illness was not viewed particularly as a priority at that time, involving carers was considered an interesting idea but not essential and interventions did not need to be seen to be evidence-based. There was no need to feel guilty about trying to be all things to all people.

CPN'd of the line?

A young man who has recently been diagnosed as having schizophrenia is discussing with his parents the prospect of returning to university to finish his degree course. Although his mother is enthusiastic, hoping he will never relapse, his father is dubious, fearing that the stress of studying will spark a second schizophrenic episode. A CPN has come to the house to give the young student his depot injection – medication that seems to keep the psychosis at bay by blocking out the voices the young man hears in his head almost every day.

It is the CPN's job to administer medication and monitor its effects, so that a balance is struck between cancelling out the disturbing auditory hallucinations without causing distressing side-effects, or adding to the lethargy that is another feature of schizophrenic illness. But it is also the CPN's job to listen to the arguments, to help the family confront the worst that might happen – relapse, acute mental illness, re-hospitalisation – and the best – survival and, perhaps, successful completion of the degree course.

Later that day the CPN may be listening to people struggling to cope with losses – bereavements, abortions, marriages dissolving, families disintegrating, or with the trauma of rape or child abuse. The CPN may be involved in teaching an agoraphobic mother how to overcome her fear of going to the local shops or perhaps helping a therapeutic group cope with a member threatening suicide.

When patients are admitted to psychiatric hospitals it can often seem as if they have been 'beamed down' like some incomprehensible alien in an old episode of *Star Trek*. But CPNs try not to view people as isolated patients with individual illnesses. Instead, they attempt to understand people suffering mental health problems within their social context – their homes, their families, their streets.

The idea of the CPN is perhaps unfamiliar to the public or, at least, not as clearly stereotyped as that of the district nurse or the health visitor. CPNs are not clearly identified with a nurse's uniform and a white cap. Indeed, they dress fairly normally. Nor do they automatically arrive, as agents of the welfare state, to perform inevitable statutory duties. Even in the history of psychiatric nursing they are a fairly new development and perhaps are still regarded by the profession and the public as an unknown quantity.

The first CPN service in Britain was started at Warlingham Park Hospital in Surrey in 1954 – relatively recently in the history of nursing. It was created partly to provide continuity of care for patients being discharged from hospital and partly because of a shortage of psychiatric social workers. These pioneering CPNs were described as 'outpatient nurses', rather than community nurses. Similarly, the only other CPN service to be established in the 1950s (at Moorhaven Hospital in Devon) was called a 'nursing after-care service'. The idea of preventing admission had not yet arrived nor, crucially, had the idea of 'community care'.

In the intervening years CPN services flourished, as outdated, long-stay institutions tried to transfer care into the community. Refinements in antipsychotic medications meant severely ill patients were more able to survive outside hospitals. CPNs rose to the challenge by becoming increasingly qualified, skilled and autonomous.

No longer are CPNs a cheap alternative to social workers nor can it be said that they are simply hospital psychiatric nurses visiting people at home. CPNs seem to be viewed with a mixture of admiration and suspicion by nursing colleagues, by doctors who once held sway over them, and by the new generation of health service managers whose managerial expertise vies for power with the CPNs' clinical expertise.

Against this background we have witnessed the rise and fall of the cult of the 'community'. Throughout the Thatcher years, working-class neighbourhoods were wracked with mass unemployment, while middle-class areas instituted 'neighbourhood watch' schemes. Mrs Thatcher suggested there was 'no such thing as society', yet the rather quaint and largely subjective notion of 'community' was enshrined in a new poll tax that was euphemistically dubbed the 'Community Charge'. Large numbers of people in this 'non-society' were unable – or unwilling – to play their full part in their 'community' by paying the charge. By the time John Major was elected they were disenfranchised along with the growing number of homeless people who share our communities.

In spite of the term 'community' having been prudently dropped from the title of the new version of the poll tax, the word lives on triumphantly in a series of White Papers, the culmination of which is the National Health Service and Community Care Act 1990. All things being equal, CPNs would have been in the vanguard of this new Act, if only by the logic of their job title. But all things are not equal. Some health authorities are now trusts and some are not. Some GPs have become fundholders and some have not. The Community Care Act gives local authorities responsibility for people with mental illnesses.

Hospital trusts and even community trusts are cropping up at a frightening rate. Many are subjecting themselves to market forces, not for the thrill of breaking free of NHS bureaucracy but out of a terrible inevitability. Likewise, multitudes of reluctant GPs are becoming fundholders.

GPs now have the power to purchase care – including mental health care – for their patients, while many trusts intend to make their money from hospitalising patients. Bang goes community care. If trusts are to make their money from admitting patients then CPNs, with their great skill in managing mental health problems in the community, are the enemy within.

It seems obvious that most people would prefer to receive treatment, care and support in their own homes, wherever possible. This is, for the most part, the 'consumer's choice'. However, under the health service reforms, the GP becomes the consumer of health care by proxy. Many GPs would acknowledge that CPNs are more knowledgeable and skilled than they are when it comes to mental health work. But, in future, they may be hampered by the demands of market forces.

CPN services could become an expensive anomaly in a highly competitive and rapidly disintegrating health care system. Alternatively, they could continue to build on their expertise and effectiveness in providing what the public wants – a comprehensive, 'user-friendly' service for a wide range of mental health problems, delivered straight to your door.

3   A day in the life – the role of the Community Psychiatric Nurse

Reflection

A good friend of mine who is a freelance journalist suggested that I ought to try my hand at writing something for a national newspaper. He told me about *The Guardian*'s regular feature, 'Diary of a . . .', and thought that they might be interested in the 'Diary of a CPN'. It was an interesting experience writing something for a general audience, rather than my usual readership of nurses and other mental health workers. On the one hand, it had to be engaging but, on the other, I was conscious of the stigma surrounding mental illness and saw this as an opportunity to educate the general public and debunk some myths. I wanted to give a flavour of a typical day without it sounding either too mundane or too sensational.

Ironically, when it was published, it carried the stand-first, 'Tony Gillam finds that even the most mundane of days can end in high drama'. In fact, a careful reading of the article shows that, while there is the potential for 'high drama' in any working day, typically most mundane days end, as might be expected, mundanely. The headline was even more ironic, suggesting great heroics on my part, which, I am sorry to say, was not the reality of the situation. 'To the rescue', it boasted. I am afraid I did not, in any literal sense, go to the rescue of any of the patients described in the article. Not the woman who had taken an overdose nor the paranoid man in the high-rise flats. 'Rescuing' is not something I go in for. Possibly, this is the whole point of 'Diary of a Community Psychiatric Nurse'.

A phrase that has stuck with me throughout my career as a CPN has been the term 'omnipotent rescuer'. This was coined, I think, by Patricia Benner and Judith Wrubel who describe it in their impressive book *The Primacy of Caring* (1989). Nurses who try to be all-powerful and to rescue patients from their predicaments may be doing so as a way of coping with their own feelings of vulnerability, because patients may leave, disappoint or die.

> The frantic rescuer who seeks to change another's behaviour as a way of gaining control and mastery may be responding to lived meanings learned early in childhood that the world is capricious and unreliable . . . the world is a risky, chaotic place that must be pasted together by one's own efforts.
>
> (Benner and Wrubel 1989: 374)

Nurses can be quick to criticise families for being 'overinvolved' with patients but may not recognise overinvolvement in themselves. It is one thing to be an autonomous practitioner and another to be, in modern parlance, a 'control freak'. Lucy Johnstone, in *Users and Abusers of Psychiatry*, borrows from the theories of Transactional Analysis to criticise the psychiatric system for playing 'the Rescue Game' with patients (Johnstone 2000).

The Rescue Game involves two players taking turns to adopt the roles of Rescuer, Persecutor and Victim. At times our patients can take on each of these roles. As mental health workers we need to avoid this situation by neither rescuing our patients, nor persecuting them, nor becoming ourselves the victims. Our job is not to rescue people, in the sense of snatching them from danger, but to quietly work with people who are at risk, who are vulnerable, to help keep them safe and well, and able to take acceptable risks in their own lives (see Chapter 5). We do this by regular visits and quiet conversation, by keeping in touch, by listening to people when they have tried to harm themselves, to help them to understand why they did it and how they could change things. We do it by supporting and supervising one another, working with families, working with groups and seeing if we can fine-tune things for people, even if we may not, personally, be able to improve their reception of Channel Five.

Diary of a Community Psychiatric Nurse

I am expecting a fairly routine Thursday. A team meeting to start the day, followed by a routine visit to a patient with schizophrenia at which I will administer his weekly injection. Then a dash back to the hospital to put in an appearance at the parasuicide team meeting in which I will describe how I assessed a young woman on a medical admissions ward who had overdosed on anti-depressants earlier that week and whether it had been appropriate to discharge her home.

Sandwiches in the car on the way to a 'clinical supervision' session with a colleague. After that, a visit to the young woman we discussed in the parasuicide meeting to find out if, at the very least, she is still alive and, at best, that the plan I proposed following her overdose enabled her to feel supported and less hopeless since I last saw her. Finally, my last visit of the day: a re-run of my first visit of the day because when I called on the patient in the morning at his brother-in-law's, as arranged, he had already caught the bus back to his own flat in the neighbouring town.

This was the day I was expecting, and it should have ended with me going back to the office to find messages from patients rearranging appointments, and letters from GPs saying: 'Could you visit this obsessional woman of 42, or this anxious young man of 17, or this young mother who is depressed because her husband blames her for his depression. . . ?' After responding to the messages and sending out appointments to all the new referrals, I would sigh at the pile of unwritten notes for all the people I had visited that day.

This was the day I was expecting but, before the meeting began at 9.30 a.m., one of my colleagues gave me a message to ring the acute psychiatric ward. When I rang the ward, the nurse said: 'We've had a phone call from the ex-girlfriend of a man who lives on the tenth floor of the high-rise flats, and he thinks that the Mafia are out to get him. Oh, and he's got a crossbow. Could you go and visit him?' So, I had to cancel the supervision session to give myself time to think about what to do about the alleged crossbow-wielding Mafia-target on the tenth floor.

As a CPN I have become desensitised to bizarre situations and absurd stories. Violence is extremely rare – I personally never use it in a professional capacity any more than my patients, who tend to be the nicest people you could wish to meet. In truth, the job of a CPN is often surprisingly neutral and lacking in high drama. Violent outbursts are rare because mentally ill people are more likely to harm themselves rather than others. I remember, when I was on call one Sunday afternoon, visiting a man who used heroin. When he unexpectedly produced a knife, he threatened to use it on himself rather than me.

The bulk of the work involves quietly listening to people talking about their worries – real or delusional – in the calm of a consulting room or, more often, in their own homes, with Jerry Springer on in the background, only interrupted by meter readers or kids coming in from school. If I want excitement it is generally up to me to create it by, for instance, training in family interventions for people with schizophrenia or co-ordinating the Music Workshop Project. This Project recently surprised us all, gaining international recognition by winning the Lilly Schizophrenia Reintegration Award. As a result, I got my picture in the local paper, which gave people something new to talk about.

One of my patients, a 59-year-old bachelor with schizophrenia, often asks me, as I am drawing up his injection, to try to adjust his TV set to see if he can get Channel Five. Last week, though, he had a different topic of conversation: 'I saw your picture in the paper, about the music you do with people with schizophrenia. Is there', he ventured, doubtfully, 'a lot of those people about then?'

Reflection

One of the striking things about psychiatric nurses is how little in common they have with nurses in general. I felt this most acutely when, as part of my basic nurse training, I was required to spend time on both medical and surgical wards. On the medical ward, my general nursing colleagues quickly identified that I was only useful for one thing – this was caring for a lady with early-onset dementia. They admitted they found her frustrating to work with and assumed that, as a *psyche nurse*, I would know how to handle her. The surgical ward was a different matter. Ruled by a cruel and tyrannical sister, the surgical ward was not a happy place for patients, relatives or staff but for psychiatric nursing students it seemed like a war zone. My general nursing colleagues found psychiatric students a strange breed. We liked to sit with patients and chat with them, rather than do things to them. I was often told off for sitting on beds. Allegedly this was to do with the risk of cross-infection but establishing a compassionate relationship with a patient seemed to be the greatest, most threatening danger.

My sister-in-law, a general nurse, had displayed a typical reaction when I announced that I was considering training as a psychiatric nurse. 'I can imagine you doing that', she said, and went on to explain that all the psychiatric nurses she had met were odd, like their patients, and had a strange sense of humour. They were also more laid-back than other nurses. I might have taken this as a discouragement, if not an insult, but I chose to take it as a valuable insight into my suitability for the job.

So, it would seem, it is helpful to be odd, laid-back and have a sense of humour. I think this is absolutely true. In fact, this may be a person-specification for prospective psychiatric nurses. To elaborate a little, we might say that it helps to be unconventional and tolerant of unconventional behaviour, that it helps to have a relaxed, liberal-minded attitude, whereby work is approached in a considered, reflective way, rather than as a series of tasks to be executed in the swiftest possible manner. A sense of humour is undoubtedly important in mental health. It might almost be said that a sense of humour represents a sense of balance and proportion and is, therefore, a hallmark of positive mental health. It is also a valuable tool in establishing therapeutic relationships with patients and in defusing anxious or emotionally charged situations.

I have observed, over the years, that psychiatric nurses have more in common with mental health workers from other disciplines, than they do with other nurses. CPNs will generally feel more at home with other mental health social workers, occupational therapists, psychiatrists and psychologists, than they will with a group of general nurses. Health visitors, midwives and practice nurses can sometimes contrive to understand psychiatric nurses, perhaps because they are fellow community workers with a certain degree of autonomy. Generally, though, 'proper' nurses react to psychiatric nurses with a mixture of bemusement and irritation. They do not understand our tolerance of strangeness, our lack of judgementalism, our 'more haste, less speed' attitude. I still feel they disapprove of me stopping to 'chat' for so long with my patients when I should be doing something!

If CPNs are laid-back, what of social workers? Everything is relative. When I undertook my diploma in community psychiatric nursing (the enigmatically titled 'ENB 812') I spent a fieldwork placement with a group of mental health social workers. I found we had a lot in common. As a CPN with psychosocial leanings, I could almost be mistaken for a social worker. I perceived the impact of society on mental health and the importance of the family. However, I was slightly envious of my social work colleagues' ability to look after themselves. Call it time management, but they sometimes let the answerphone kick in instead of rushing to answer a call when they were in mid-conversation. Call it caseload management, but they seemed to have fewer people to worry about than me. I was privileged to be able to visit clients and see assessments conducted from a social work perspective. I also conducted semi-structured interviews with social workers about the differences between community psychiatric nursing and mental health social work. All this reinforced the impressions I had gained from experience and from the literature. Differences in individual personality are more important than differences in training or professional practice.

The common task of working with stigmatised people – mentally ill people – can unite mental health workers from any discipline. We are stigmatised ourselves by our peculiar decision to choose to work with the mentally ill. Workers in the field of physical health see mental health as 'something else', not real illness, not real nursing. Much more discussion needs to take place about the role of mental health workers in the community, whatever discipline we may call ourselves. The thrust towards multi-disciplinary training and multi-disciplinary work is to be welcomed as we forge new identities for ourselves.

The role of community mental health workers

There would appear to be several areas of overlap between the work of the mental health social worker (MHSW) and that of the CPN. These similarities raise questions about how work in community mental health should be divided among various members of the multi-disciplinary team in order to make best use of available resources. Differences in client group, operational base, size of team, the perceptions of the professionals themselves, their colleagues and the public are all likely to influence the service delivered. Furthermore, differences in training and culture are likely to influence the ideological bases of the two groups while, in turn, ideology may affect styles of working.

While there is a growing body of literature concerning both mental health social work and community psychiatric nursing as separate entities, there is little direct comparison between the two groups. It, therefore, seems important to explore and describe some areas of convergence and divergence.

Mental health social work is a specialised area of social work, while community psychiatric nursing has been described as 'a sub-division of psychiatric nursing which is itself a speciality within the occupational category of "nursing"' (Morrall 1989: 7). Given that both are examples of specialities arising relatively recently out of two professions, some discussion of the historical development of the two groups seems necessary.

The origins of CPN services in Britain are inextricably linked with the social work profession. The first CPN services in the 1950s were created partly because of a shortage of what were then referred to as psychiatric social workers (May and Moore 1963). From these 'after-care' services for the chronically mentally ill, community psychiatric nursing developed, so that, by the 1960s, some services were operating from general practices or health centres.

Concepts of 'community care' and 'community psychiatry' emerged, alongside a movement for care and treatment away from mental hospitals. It might have been expected that 'mental welfare officers' or 'psychiatric social workers' would have played a central role in this movement but by the early 1970s the reorganisation of social services in the wake of the *Seebohm Report* (DHSS 1968) had led to the disappearance of these specialist mental health social workers.

In their place, local authorities had established social services departments wherein 'generic' social workers divided their time between a variety of client groups. It has been suggested that:

> these personnel were unable to gain sufficient experience with the mentally ill . . . and lacked any special training in such work. This process further encouraged the development of CPN services because of the gap that had developed in the care of psychiatric patients outside hospital at a time when increasing numbers . . . were being discharged.
>
> (Rawlinson and Brown 1991)

This shift to genericism in social work has since been countered by the Mental Health Act 1983 which, once again, established specialist MHSWs (approved social workers). The resulting coexistence of both CPN services and MHSW services in many areas raises a number of questions about an overlap of roles.

Given the historical context, comparisons between the two groups are perhaps inevitable. Griffith and Mangen, in discussing the role definition of the CPN, noted: 'There was considerable overlap in performance with district nurse, health visitors and social workers. Roles were undifferentiated since they were all working towards the common goal of helping patients with emotional difficulties' (Griffith and Mangen 1980: 203). In reviewing the literature, these authors found a general belief that 'psychiatric nurses had a distinct advantage in dealing with the mentally ill in the community . . . because of their basic psychiatric skills, psychiatric nurses were better prepared to identify and deal with psychiatric syndromes at the acute stage' (ibid.).

While there can be little doubt that psychiatric nurses are more skilled than other nurses in dealing with acute psychiatric syndromes, the question of the relative effectiveness of specialist MHSWs is debatable. Writing before the inception of the Mental Health Act 1983, Griffith and Mangen could only observe that:

> The abolition of the role of psychiatric social workers to generic social workers as recommended in the [*Seebohm Report*] . . . resulted in

increased contributions of psychiatric nurses to the domiciliary treatment service. Psychiatric nursing began to develop a more differentiated role in terms of making definite contributions to the treatment of patients in the community.

(ibid.)

They also noted the trend for CPNs to take a more social, environmental and interpersonal approach, thus shifting from a narrow medical model to a quasi-social work model.

One example of the CPN as MHSW is given by Sladden in a contemporaneous book devoted to psychiatric nursing in the community (Sladden 1979). She delineates five functions of the CPN – clinical, psychosocial, environmental, internal liaison and external liaison. Only the first of these is unique to the CPN, that is, the observation of clinical signs and side-effects, the administration of medication and the regulation of treatment regimes. This clinical function includes what Sladden (perhaps ironically) referred to as the main raison d'être of CPNs – the administration of depot injections. It also includes carrying out psychiatric assessment on behalf of doctors and guidance on clinical management to GPs, health visitors, district nurses and others.

The remaining four functions of the CPN include areas traditionally associated with social work, such as psychotherapy (individual, family and conjoint work), group work (especially away from the hospital), anxiety management, social skills training, home assessment, environmental support (for example, enlisting home help or meals-on-wheels services), helping with accommodation problems, liaising between the psychiatric team and primary care teams, and providing back-up and advice to voluntary groups and self-help groups. If the CPN can do all this, on top of a clinical role, it could be argued that there is little need for specialist MHSWs. This conclusion led Griffith and Mangen to urge a close examination of the overlapping of roles 'so as to eliminate role conflict which may result from duplication of roles' (Griffith and Mangen 1980: 206). Just such a close examination began in the wake of the Mental Health Act 1983. With the re-emergence of specialist MHSWs having statutory duties (as Approved Social Workers or ASWs), the role overlap debate gathered momentum.

Wooff *et al.* compared the practice of community psychiatric nursing and mental health social work in Salford (Wooff *et al.* 1988; Wooff and Goldberg 1988). Although they found some overlap between the two groups, significant differences emerged. First, they found that the CPNs tended to focus on psychiatric symptoms, treatment and medication far more than the social workers in the study. This is not surprising, given the CPN's 'clinical function' described above. The social workers dealt with a wider range of topics and were as concerned with social interactions and with family and community networks as with individual symptoms. This might suggest that, despite Sladden's five-function model, MHSWs were, after all, better at social work than CPNs.

Second, the study found that CPNs spent less time with psychotic clients than with neurotic ones, compared with the MHSWs, who spent a similar amount of time with both. More alarmingly, this suggests that not only are MHSWs better at social work but that CPNs cannot claim a monopoly of commitment to the severely mentally ill.

A third finding was that CPNs had less contact with other members of the mental health team and more with the primary care team. This is partly a matter of geography. In the Salford study, CPNs were community-based, MHSWs hospital-based. It could be argued that this is atypical; while less than half of CPN teams are based in hospitals, MHSWs being hospital-based is the exception rather than the rule (White 1990). Where CPNs did have contact with the mental health team, this was, not surprisingly, predominantly with a psychiatrist.

Finally, Wooff *et al.* found that when working with non-schizophrenic clients, CPNs were more likely to show disapproval or to be directive than MHSWs. They were also more likely to undertake physical or behavioural treatments.

Rawlinson and Brown saw the findings of Wooff *et al.* as supporting the notion that CPNs are inadequately trained (Rawlinson and Brown 1991) just as Skidmore and Friend had found (Skidmore and Friend 1984). Rawlinson and Brown suggested, however, that this 'skills deficit' allegedly found among CPNs could change with the gradual appearance of nurses trained under the 1982 Registered Mental Nurse (RMN) syllabus. This placed a greater emphasis on both individual skills and community care and aimed to provide 'a relevant preparation for the mental nurse to enable practice in the hospital or community setting' (ENB 1987).

So while Griffith and Mangen considered the CPN to have 'a distinct advantage' and Sladden implied that the CPN's role largely absorbed that of the MHSW, Wooff *et al.* found CPNs less effective than MHSWs, and Rawlinson and Brown concluded they were inadequately trained. Can this really be the case, when CPNs have at least three years' specialist training, compared with the MHSWs' generic and usually shorter training?

Huxley is less positive about social workers, stating that they 'do not recognise much of the psychological disorder presented to them and do not act upon it – either on their own or in concert with others' (Huxley 1991). He went on to complain that 'social workers contrive to assume that they are the "only" defenders of patient/client rights, to the annoyance of other disciplines who argue that they, too, have this responsibility' (ibid.). He noted that social workers outside hospitals (and this, of course, excludes those in the Salford study) were reluctant to accept medical referral for fear of encouraging the 'medical auxiliary' view of their profession.

Just as CPNs' skills may have been enhanced by the 1982 syllabus, the Mental Health Act 1983 may have changed social work's relationship to medicine, since ASWs now have a clear responsibility to take medical opinion into account when forming an independent opinion about the hospitalisation of clients. Huxley also felt that MHSWs' competence might have been improved by the introduction of ASW training courses. Before the 1983 Act, according to Huxley, more than half of the trained social workers in the UK had less than five hours' specific training in psychiatry (ibid.).

Huxley argued that great variations within professional groups indicated that 'personal perspectives may override professional conformity' (ibid.). This is in agreement with Horder, who sweepingly stated: 'Job descriptions, separate trainings, and professional boundaries are of no importance; what counts is the personality, understanding and behaviour of the individual worker' (Horder 1986). Horder compared doctors with social workers and found glaring differences in their views on cases of depression. While the social workers thought the doctors were overly concerned with diagnostic labelling and too ready to use drugs as treatment, doctors found social workers reluctant to recognise non-social causes of depression.

Jefferys also wrote about social work's relation to medicine (Jefferys 1986). The *Seebohm Report*, according to Jefferys, had successfully ended social work's subordination to the medical profession so that, even where social workers work in NHS hospitals or GP units, they do so as seconded staff with responsibility to the local authority rather than to a doctor. She noted, however, that the rapid expansion post-Seebohm was only made possible by recruiting many young, untrained social workers. Along with Huxley's earlier comment about five hours' psychiatric training, this may explain the belief, held by many GPs, that a social worker's skills in psychotherapy were no greater than their own (ibid.).

Despite Wooff's work, it seems doctors are reluctant to share power and responsibility with social workers. There are cultural differences between the professions that exacerbate this situation. Clare and Corney report doctors' 'frustration concerning the paucity of information fed back to them from social workers to whom they have referred patients' (Clare and Corney 1982).

Another source of friction, quite apart from the sometimes unpopular decisions social workers make, is the time they take to make them:

> Differences in working tempo are a particular problem. Doctors often become impatient when immediate action is not taken by social workers to alleviate difficulties, whereas the social worker, trained to take a more long-term perspective, sited within a complex and often slow-moving bureaucracy, and answerable to administrative supervisors, can rarely take decisions with quite the same degree of facility.
>
> (ibid.)

It is interesting to juxtapose this last point with the concept of crisis intervention wherein 'the CPN is often the most flexible member of the team, able to respond to a crisis situation early' (Rawlinson and Brown 1991). Thus, speed of intervention would seem one of the advantages CPNs have over MHSWs but might also account for Wooff and colleagues' findings that

CPNs spend less time with psychotic patients and tend to be more directive with non-schizophrenic patients.

Clare and Corney observed that some social workers regarded psychoanalytically derived approaches to psychologically disturbed people as 'the definitive treatment modality'. At the same time, they were often 'ignorant about the use of medication in conditions such as schizophrenia'. They were also uncertain of the value of maintenance medication and unclear about the distinctions and similarities between the side-effects of such medication and symptoms of the original illness (Clare and Corney 1982). It is debatable whether this confusion about medication is due to lack of training, anti-psychiatry ideology or the slower decision-making process mentioned above.

A review of the literature provides a mixed picture. The bulk of material on the subject is conceptual in nature and explores subjective experiences of the work of CPNs and MHSWs, often from the point of view of other professionals, particularly doctors.

The work of Wooff *et al.* stands out as one of the few relevant studies with an experimental design. It is of its time, in that the effects of the Mental Health Act 1983 are obvious and changes to the RMN syllabus (1982) were beginning to filter through. Strangely, though, a decade after the *Seebohm Report* had shifted most social workers away from the hospital, those in this study were well integrated into the hospital team. By contrast, CPNs in the study were primary care-based and extremely isolated from the psychiatric team, at a time when many were still not even open to GP referrals. Wooff *et al.* concede that 'the Salford services may not be . . . typical of others' (Wooff *et al.* 1988: 790; Wooff and Goldberg 1988).

With little beyond conceptual material to review, it is hard to draw any firm conclusions about the differences and similarities between CPNs and MHSWs. Overall, however, the literature would suggest that Huxley is right to argue that 'personal perspectives may override professional conformity' (Huxley 1991).

4 Learning in lay-bys
Teaching and assessing

Reflection

The idea of reflective practice underpins this book. Although always given to reflection, it was not until I undertook a course on teaching and assessing that I started giving serious consideration to the concept of the reflective practitioner. The course, affectionately known as 'ENB 998', is extremely popular with nurses because this qualification is traditionally considered 'desirable', if not 'essential', in any number of advertisements for jobs.

To give it its proper title, ENB 997/998 (Teaching and Assessing in Clinical Practice) varies a great deal in duration from one area to another. In some places it can involve up to six months of part-time study, in other places only a few days. Although, at times, a bit too involved and intensive for my liking, I can at least say that the course I did gave me a good grounding in some of the key issues concerning teaching and learning, assessing, mentoring, preceptorship and reflective practice.

What is reflective practice? At its worst, it can seem like another of those fads, yet another requirement of the nursing establishment, and something that nurses have to dutifully inflict upon themselves. It is this tendency that Bowles (1995) pokes fun at, when he writes of the reluctance of the nursing profession – in the UK especially – 'to approach the serious business of nursing with anything less than scientific or academically acceptable labels' (Bowles 1995: 366). I was intrigued, though, when I came across his idea of using 'story-telling' as a way of enriching nurses' lives. After all, it is the wealth of fascinating human stories that makes psychiatric nursing such an interesting job.

Nurses do tell stories, in their reflective diaries, in professional portfolios, in case studies and in clinical supervision, and it is not that these forms of reflection are bad in themselves. (Indeed, Chapter 5 goes on to describe the benefits of supervision while Chapter 10 shows how case studies can be used to improve patient care and make us feel more positive about our nursing practice.) There is nothing wrong with these tools for reflection but Bowles is critical of 'the attendant jargon and models for implementation' with which we make things more difficult for ourselves (ibid.).

It is not only nurses who desiccate the stories that are at the heart of our work. The neurologist and author Oliver Sacks writes of how neurologists and psychiatrists have lost the art of powerful description (Sacks 1986). Hippocrates introduced the 'case history' (a description, or depiction, of the natural history of disease) but Sacks argues that:

> there is no 'subject' in a narrow case history; modern case histories allude to the subject in a cursory phrase ('a trisomic albino female of 21'), which could as well apply to a rat as a human being. To restore the human subject at the centre . . . we must deepen a case history to a narrative or tale: only then do we have a 'who' as well as a 'what'.
>
> (Sacks 1986: x)

Of course, in reflective writing on psychiatric nursing it is not just the 'what' of the disease that can obscure the 'who' of the patient but the 'what' of the nursing that can obscure the 'who' of the nurse.

It is worthwhile, then, to combine the thinking of both Sacks and Bowles when considering how reflective practice can inform teaching and learning. Sacks urges us to 'deepen' our case histories to restore the human subject to the centre of the story (ibid.). Bowles believes that story-telling is capable of effecting personal change in the narrator as well as the audience and that it can mitigate the loss of identity, and the impoverishment of role models and collegial networks (Bowles 1995).

It follows from this that CPNs can use story-telling to enrich their practice. We should tell stories, about our patients, about our work, in our reflective diaries, in professional portfolios, in clinical supervision and, of course, in everyday conversation with each other. Perhaps we should also develop what Bowles calls our 'collegial network' by writing more stories, as case studies, articles and books, which have a 'who' as well as a 'what'.

Teaching and learning in lay-bys – applying reflective practice to teaching in the community

I first heard the term 'parking in lay-bys' used in an education context while on a course on teaching and learning in clinical practice (ENB 997/998). The phrase was being used metaphorically, of course, in the sense that, sometimes in the course of their practice, nurses need to 'pull over' and reflect on what they do, before continuing on their journey.

The idea struck a particular chord with me since I had become aware that, as a CPN, I quite often *literally* parked in lay-bys, in order to reflect upon the previous, or next, visit to a patient. I sometimes use time between visits to write notes, dictate clinical letters or simply reflect on my work. I am in the habit of using the car as a mobile office so that, whenever I find a patient not at home, I am able to make use of the time.

CPN placements are always popular with learners of all kinds. Apart from pre-registration students on extended placements, it is common for CPNs to be asked to 'give a day out' to enrolled nurses on conversion courses, 'Return to Nursing' students, as well as trainee doctors, social workers and psychologists. These learners nearly always have lots of questions about interventions used in psychiatric nursing, the medication used and current legislation. Inevitably, CPNs find themselves discussing, teaching, reflecting and supervising, while we drive from one patient to another. While advocates of road safety may not approve, I would argue that what might be termed 'teach as we go' along with the 'parking in lay-bys' method of learning have much to commend them.

The '998' course involves planning, implementing and evaluating a number of teaching sessions. Four of my six formative teaching sessions took the form of impromptu lessons. Three of these were 'in-car' sessions, covering topics such as policies and procedures in the CPN department, the Care Programme Approach, the Supervision Register, Supervised Discharge and the art of giving depot injections in the community. These topics arose naturally out of the preoccupations of the student involved. The subject matter was of unquestionable value: case management of people with severe mental illness, along with consideration of their medication needs. Gournay stresses the importance of case management and underlines that, although 'recent years have seen the emergence of important psychosocial interventions . . . the issue of medication and its management remains arguably the priority for clients with the most severe problems' (Gournay 1995: 12).

If the content of my 'lay-by' teaching sessions was highly relevant, what of the method? It could be argued that the 'lay-by' teaching session is a perfect illustration of experiential learning in that, according to Merchant, it 'begins with experience' (interacting with patients) 'which is followed by reflection, discussion, analysis and evaluation of the experience' (in my case debriefing in the car). 'This leads to understanding that is meaningful for the individual. The other key feature is that it is always done by the learner sorting things out for himself' (Merchant 1989: 308).

Experiential learning is closely related to the concept of andragogy, the key elements of which are summarised by Milligan:

> facilitation of adult learning that can best be achieved through a student-centred approach that, in a developmental manner, enhances the student's self-concept, promotes autonomy, self-direction and critical thinking, reflects on experience and involves the learner in the diagnosis, planning, enaction and evaluation of their own learning needs.
>
> (Milligan 1995: 22)

This description of andragogy can be juxtaposed with Merchant's comment that experiential learning 'requires that the individual deals with real problems' (Merchant 1989: 308). It seems reasonable to argue, then, that the philosophy of andragogy coupled with the methods of experiential learning are congruent with the aims of educating students in the field of community psychiatric nursing.

If methodology and choice of subject seem appropriate, impromptu teaching sessions could still be criticised were they to represent the sole teaching strategy of the CPN. The strengths of impromptu sessions seem to be immediacy, spontaneity and the instant addressing of learning needs. There is little risk of material being mismatched with the needs or level of the learners because they – not the teacher – decide these. The weakness of impromptu teaching lies in the lack of opportunity for lengthy reflection prior to teaching and the lack of preparation of materials that might aid or consolidate learning. There is also a more general criticism of student-centred learning, enunciated by Burnard (1989), which is

> a question of developing a balance between what Heron (1986) calls 'following' and 'leading'. Following involves taking the lead from students, using their experience and ideas. Leading, on the other hand, means making suggestions and using structure to help the students. . . . Having said this, the attitude towards nurse education should always remain student-centred.
>
> (Burnard 1989: 304)

The need for uniting these methods, which, according to Burnard, ensures balance and symmetry, is astutely satisfied in my own particular clinical area by the CPN department's 'educational sessions'. The educational session is a monthly meeting of 60 or 90 minutes' duration, which is pre-arranged to meet the learning needs and interests of the CPN team. Student nurses on placement in the department are encouraged to attend these sessions, although the primary aim is the in-service development of practising CPNs. Over the last five years my colleagues and I have been involved with organising these sessions and we have also undertaken some of the teaching.

The CPN educational meeting can be seen as an 'ideal' teaching forum, in that it ensures a dedicated period of time and an almost guaranteed audience. It allows for careful preparation of the session, with pre-planning of aims and objectives, method of teaching, materials needed and the opportunity for feedback or evaluation of the session. It could almost be said that, in its capacity for formal structure, it is a compensation for the informed improvisation (that is, parking in lay-bys), which constitutes the typical CPN teaching and learning experience.

If the planned CPN educational meeting allows for far greater preparation and structure, this does not mean that it needs to make use of didactic, teacher-centred methods. As Burnard has said, 'the attitude to nurse education should always remain student-centred' (Burnard 1989: 304). Since undertaking the '998' course, I have come to realise, more and more, that the CPN educational session provides an opportunity to *expand* upon topics and themes that arise naturally in discussion with colleagues and which, often, will have been the subject of impromptu teaching. Thus, for example, following an initial meeting with a colleague to whom I was asked to be preceptor, I identified some confusion about the terms preceptor, mentor and clinical supervision. On the basis of this, I planned a formal teaching session on preceptorship in mental health, aiming to clear up these confusions. This session was 'slotted' into the CPN educational meeting and formed one of my summative assessments for the course. It was attended by several CPNs, including two who were undergoing preceptorship and one (in addition to myself) who was acting as a preceptor.

Being able to facilitate learning in the CPN department, then, hinges on a combination of two teaching strategies. The first of these is impromptu teaching, what I have called 'teach as you go' or 'parking in lay-bys'. The second strategy involves utilising the regular CPN educational meetings as a forum for more structured sessions, which may develop themes from the impromptu teaching.

It should be remembered that the phrase 'parking in lay-bys' was used, not with reference to a teaching strategy but, metaphorically, to denote a way of considering reflective practice. Much has been written in the nursing literature about reflective practice (and, indeed, it is the unifying concept behind this book). The need for reflection in nursing (and, I would argue, also in teaching) has arisen because of what can be viewed as an overemphasis on science, measurable outcomes, behavioural 'competences' and market forces, along with the devaluing of andragogy, humanism and the artistic elements in nursing (Burrows 1995; Milligan 1995; Bowles 1995).

Burrows discusses how 'nursing education creates a narrow interpretation of critical thinking as a linear problem-solving system . . . with students expected to utilise research-based theory in a logical systematic manner in order to achieve certain practical competencies' (Burrows 1995: 346). The 'back to basics' climate of recent years has put andragogy and experiential learning under siege. Burrows lamented that 'in both nursing and the scientific method, knowledge derived from practice tends to be undervalued' and he argues that 'critical thinking should be grounded in reflecting upon both experience and knowledge. By acknowledging the value of such learning, nursing may come to appreciate the potential benefits to the client of bringing together its scientific and artistic elements' (ibid.).

This seems to be a plea for a return to more humanistic values in nursing. It might even be suspected that some of the remaining exponents of andragogy and experiential learning are about to 'hijack' reflective practice as a last bastion. If this were so, it would not be without irony that an edict from the United Kingdom Central Council (UKCC) could become the saving grace of the art of nursing, for it was the UKCC that prescribed nurses should be 'able to think critically' (UKCC 1986).

Bowles has the perfect antidote to all 'the confusing and almost elitist rhetoric which surrounds reflective practice' (Bowles 1995: 368). He searches for meaning in story-telling and notes that, in contrast to the wealth of literature from the United States about the use of story-telling in nursing, there is almost a complete lack of it in the British literature. 'This may be indicative', he suggests, 'of a degree of reticence in the UK to approach the serious business of nursing with anything less than scientific or academically acceptable labels' (ibid.). British nurses do tell stories in reflective diaries, professional portfolios, case studies and clinical supervision but, Bowles feels, 'the contrast between these narrow "reflective" techniques (and the attendant jargon and models for implementation) and the apparent simplicity of telling stories is clearly apparent' (ibid.).

Great use is made of people's stories in my own CPN department. For instance, GPs send us referral letters that tell the story of how a patient has come to need our help, following which we go to assess patients and invite them to tell their own story. In discussing the patients in reviews and in clinical supervision sessions we retell these stories, and in writing care plans, nursing notes and discharge summaries of patients we recount the story of our intervention and its outcome. In these ways we validate our work, share our insights, develop our professionalism and provide paradigms from which our colleagues can learn.

Bowles suggests that story-telling 'is a medium by which personal experience can be communicated to others with immediacy and relevancy and which is capable of effecting personal change in the *narrator* as well as the audience' (Bowles 1995: 366). He also believes that the 'loss of identity, and the impoverishment of role models and collegial networks may be mitigated by story telling' (ibid.).

One of the earliest influences on my thoughts about teaching and learning came from a collection of stories called *How Children Fail* (Holt 1969). I read this – essentially the reflective journal of an American schoolteacher – the year I left school and went to university (the year I left a pedagogical institution for an andragogical one). Two years after that, I found myself teaching French children to speak English in a school in Brittany. There, still under the spell of John Holt, I kept my own reflective notes on my classroom experiences.

Despite a fiercely experiential, andragogical nurse training – thanks to the influence of the 1982 syllabus (ENB 1982) – my ten years of nursing have not been untouched by 'the Post-Thatcherite Philistine Hurricane' (Milligan 1995: 25). Perhaps it took the ENB 997/998 course, with all its talk of competences, learning objectives and performance criteria, to rouse me from my post-Thatcherite sleep.

The need for a resurgence in the primacy of andragogy and experiential learning, along with reflective practice, is long overdue. Milligan reminds us that 'we must be politically aware and active in our defence of educational methods that we find useful and appropriate, yet are politically unfashionable or perhaps too challenging in the wider socio-economic context' (ibid.).

As regards the CPN department, it would seem that a combination of impromptu teaching and more formally prepared sessions within a programme of educational meetings is a valid and highly relevant means of facilitating learning. This learning, however, needs also to take place within a culture of reflective practice. For some, compiling reflective journals may promote this but in this article the imaginative use of story-telling has been explored. The value of stories, according to Bowles (1995), is that they contextualise and humanise knowledge and deal with the 'know-how' of nursing, which Benner (1984) identifies as being essential to skilled practice.

New perspectives are more valuable to nurses and to teachers than any 'essential' knowledge. As my first mentor, John Holt, wrote:

> We cannot possibly judge what knowledge will be most needed forty, or twenty, or even ten years from now. . . . It is not subject matter that makes some learning more valuable than others, but the spirit in which the work is done.
>
> (Holt 1969: 173–4)

Reflection

While teaching and learning in lay-bys can be fun, assessing sounds an altogether different sort of business. Assessing, in the sense of assessing nursing students' abilities, has, for me, less positive connotations. Words like 'policing' and 'gate-keeping' come to mind. Teaching and learning are necessary but often enjoyable, whereas assessment seems like a serious business, a necessary evil.

Why does assessing students seem so different to assessing patients? An assessment of a patient is often the springboard, the start of a therapeutic relationship that may last for weeks or years but is the beginning of a journey taken together. Despite any amount of talk about continuous assessment, or even 'summative' and 'formative' assessments, I get the impression that many nursing students still see the assessment process as something coming at the end of an episode of learning, almost like a driving test. Can they drive or not? Can they nurse or not?

I prefer to view assessment as part of a continuous process of learning, practice, evaluation and reflection, which I, as a reflective, practising CPN, am experiencing as much as any student. If students reduce my perhaps rather noble conception of the situation to a case of 'Have I done well enough, or not?' then this is a cultural problem.

My article, 'Taking a humanistic approach to assessment', was written partly as a revolt against the prevailing culture in nurse education. It seemed to me that the art of psychiatric nursing was in danger of being reduced to a series of 'tick boxes' called, in the jargon of the ENB, 'competences' or, in that of the UKCC, 'outcomes'. In the mid-1990s it was not difficult to imagine (or recognise, depending on your point of view) that a conspiracy was being perpetrated upon the public sector. Health and welfare, education, the arts, were being circumscribed by narrow rules and regulations, outcome measures, league tables and guidelines. A wonderful phrase quoted by Milligan (1995), which is attributed to *The Guardian* newspaper, suggested that we were living in the wake of the 'Post-Thatcherite Philistine Hurricane'. The effect of this on what I had always considered to be essentially humanistic, creative activities, like nursing and teaching, was rather like a return to the utilitarianism of Victorian times. Utilitarianism was a school of moral philosophy, originally proposed by Jeremy Bentham and John Stuart Mill, that held that all moral, social or political action should be directed towards the greatest good for the greatest number of people. At its most basic, utilitarianism argues that what is useful is good. Dickens brilliantly lampooned the theory in his novel *Hard Times*: 'Now, what I want is Facts. Teach these boys and girls nothing but Facts. Facts alone are wanted in life. . . . This is the principle on which I bring up these children. Stick to Facts, sir!' (Dickens 1854: 47). This is Mr Gradgrind advising the schoolmaster on how to teach the children according to his own narrow, utilitarian beliefs. Dickens continues:

> No little Gradgrind had ever associated a cow in a field with that famous cow with the crumpled horn who tossed the dog who worried the cat who killed the rat who ate the malt, or with that yet more famous cow who swallowed Tom Thumb: it had never heard of those celebrities, and had only been introduced to a cow as a gramnivorous ruminating quadruped with several stomachs. . . .
>
> (Dickens 1854: 54)

We would do well to be aware of utilitarianism in the field of mental health. We would do well to be aware of reductionism of any sort, and this is the argument underpinning 'Taking a humanistic approach to assessment'.

At the time of writing, in the wake of that 'Post-Thatcherite Philistine Hurricane', it seemed to me that reductionism, utilitarianism, Thatcherism and behaviourism were all part of the same thing. My views on this have changed somewhat since undertaking training in behavioural family therapy and seeing the benefits of this in practice with the families of people with schizophrenia (see Chapter 10). I think behavioural approaches, focusing on what people do, need not be reductionist or dehumanising as long as they are grounded in a person-centred, humanistic approach. If our nursing practice should be patient-centred and our teaching learner-centred, then it follows that our assessment process, even if it must perform a policing, gate-keeping function, must be student-centred. Not in a narrow way that concerns itself only with this or that competency but as part of the process of developing skills, knowledge and insight integral to the lifelong evolution of reflective practitioners.

Taking a humanistic approach to assessment – the assessment of nursing competence in the community

Nursing is a profession bounded by rules, regulations, guidelines, recommendations, codes of conduct and practice, national boards and a central council. Within the profession, as Young points out:

> the traditional approach to teaching and assessing has been to impose a clearly defined body of knowledge and practical expertise on the student which is then assessed in a somewhat impersonal and authoritarian manner. The hierarchical structure of the nursing profession tends to perpetuate such methods and attitudes and in spite of changing techniques, the power is seen to be firmly in the hands of the teacher and assessor.
>
> (Young 1994)

Although the CPN is likely to work in a less hierarchical setting and is less likely to be 'impersonal and authoritarian', this power differential still undeniably exists. Merchant makes the point that 'because the current assessment system leads to professional qualification the livelihood of the individual is dependent upon the results' (Merchant 1989: 311).

However, the key feature of assessment seems to hinge on the measuring of 'competence'. For example, Everett defines an assessor as one who has 'responsibility to ensure professional competence is achieved by the student nurse' (Everett 1995: 8). The assessor is thus 'accountable both to the learner, in giving fair judgement, and to the public in ensuring the standards of professional competence are achieved' (ibid.). As such, the nurse who is an assessor stands between the student nurse with his or her ambition to qualify as a practitioner and the freedom to practise. It could be argued that this 'gate-keeping' role is obstructive rather than facilitative or, at least, inherently conservative. Young underlines this when she writes:

> There are a number of legal implications for employer, teacher, assessor and learner in the performance of their roles. On the whole the law is concerned with ensuring safety of the patient and the rights of the student must be secondary.
>
> (Young 1994: 169)

There might seem to be, then, a conflict between the assessor's role (which is ultimately to protect patients and uphold professional standards) and that of the mentor, whose allegiance might appear to be to the student. The English National Board has defined 'mentor' as one who 'by example and facilitation, guides, assists and supports the student in new learning skills, adopting new behaviours and acquiring new attitudes' (Young 1994: 161). However, the same glossary definition stipulates that the term 'mentor' refers to 'an appropriately qualified and experienced first level nurse' (ibid.). As such, the mentor cannot be someone who puts a learner's needs or rights above the needs or rights of patients since, by definition, a nurse's first duty is to the patient.

Some of these tensions might be overcome by splitting the roles of mentor and assessor between two qualified nurses. This has advantages: the mentor and the assessor can compare notes on the learner's progress and this can lead to greater objectivity. The learner cannot blame a 'personality clash' in the event of a poor report but, on the negative side, the learner may feel victimised by any perceived 'conspiracy' between mentor and assessor. The greatest disadvantage, however, may be the doubling of staff time where mentor and assessor are not one and the same person. Qualified staff and their managers may not consider this a cost-effective use of resources.

Returning to the difficulty of assessing competence in community psychiatric nursing, it may be helpful to illustrate this with an example from clinical practice. A third-year student on placement in a CPN department needs to be assessed on his or her counselling skills. This commonplace scenario raises several interesting points. The essential areas of clinical competence to be measured in community psychiatric nursing typically involve interpersonal skills. It can be difficult to measure these skills objectively and precisely since they depend on abstract qualities (e.g. empathy, warmth, genuineness), and on the patient's subjective experience of the counselling relationship. Burnard makes the point that, in reflecting on such personal qualities in counselling, there is an assumption 'that we are all in agreement about what constitutes "warmth", "empathy" and so on'. Burnard questions the soundness of this assumption, suggesting 'it might be argued that one person's "warmth" is another person's "sickliness"' (Burnard 1994). There is likely to be far less disagreement, for example, about the materials needed to carry out an accurate test of a patient's urine.

So, assessment tools that might be sufficient to assess more concrete, practical nursing skills (e.g. urine testing) are likely to be too unsophisticated to be of use. Judgements about use of equipment and using the *correct* procedure can become absurdly inappropriate. There are few absolutes in community psychiatric nursing; rarely is there a right and wrong way to intervene. However, a skilled CPN is able to make judgements about whether the student's approach and style of intervention is likely to be more or less helpful to the patient. This, however, would seem not to be enough since the assessor needs to make an absolute judgement about whether or not the student is competent.

Even the abstract, qualitative notion of competence has become a concrete, quantifiable item. The dictionary defines competence as 'the state or *quality* of being capable or competent' (Reader's Digest 1987: 326). The English National Board, however, has made competence 'the ability to perform a *particular* activity *to a prescribed standard*' (Young 1994: 161). This obsession with measuring competence can be viewed as symptomatic of the political climate of the last two decades, which is persecuting the art of nursing along with other educational and welfare services. Milligan dramatised this when he wrote that:

> We live in the wake of the 'Post-Thatcherite Philistine Hurricane' [a term first used by *The Guardian* newspaper], an era that devalued . . . the arts and more liberal forms of education. There were, of course, the persistent references to 'Back to Basics', which in educational terms seemed to imply a move away from radical/liberal educational methods.
>
> (Milligan 1995: 25)

Milligan goes on to make reference to 'the strict control of curriculum content achieved through the National Curriculum and the assessments that go with it [which] mitigate against recent moves towards a more student-centred approach' (ibid.).

If centralised curricular control and 'back to basics' ideology have held sway in all fields of education, it could be argued that nurse education is no exception. Nursing curricula have dutifully been redesigned to fit with the 'competences', reducing nurse education to a process of jumping through hurdles dressed up as student-centred, experiential, adult learning. 'The emphasis on defined outcomes, as opposed to educational process', writes Milligan, 'is perhaps a manifestation of the institutionalised ideology of behaviourism' (ibid.). He argues that 'the definition of competence' [the attainment of which is the primary aim of assessment] 'has been adversely influenced by a behaviourist approach', which Milligan (along with Ashworth and Morrison) suggests had been broadly encouraged by the then recently deposed Conservative Government (Milligan 1995; Ashworth and Morrison 1991).

All this perhaps smacks too much of conspiracy theory and might be dismissed as no more than the paranoia of the hitherto disenfranchised British Left. Bowles (1995), however, draws on American sources, to argue in a similar vein that current concepts of assessment – and particularly competence in its new sense – have led to a 'sense of impoverishment of human values' (Sarosi and O'Connor 1993). Bowles asserts that 'the introduction of the free market in the NHS has subjected nurses to an increasingly scientific style of management in which skill mix and *psychomotor competencies* are linguistic symbols of a reductionist new order' (Bowles 1995: 366). The assessment of psychomotor competencies, then, is seen as part of a process that is leading to a loss of meaning in the nursing profession.

The term 'assessment process', in the light of such arguments, takes on an overtone: ironic, mocking, even sinister. 'The value of *process* in education' which, Milligan reminds us, is an integral part of andragogy (see below), 'is rather clouded when comments from the United Kingdom Central Council (UKCC) are examined – "*Today's rules are concerned with outcomes*, not with the process by which those outcomes are to be achieved" [UKCC 1986, original emphasis]. Such a view is inconsistent with the promotion of andragogy as published the following year by the ENB' (Milligan 1995: 26; UKCC 1986; ENB 1987).

Andragogy is a concept worthy of further elaboration. It describes an approach to the theory and practice of adult education once lauded within nurse education and now, as Milligan implies (above), somewhat beleaguered. Burnard (1989) provides a useful summary of andragogy's basic tenets (see Table 4.1).

Table 4.1 Burnard's summary of andragogy (or adult education) (adapted from Burnard (1989))

1. Adult education should be grounded in the participants' wealth of prior experience
2. Adults need to be able to apply what they learn
3. Adult education should be an active rather than a passive process
4. In common with many experiential learning approaches, andragogy emphasises the centrality of personal experience and subjective interpretation

To suggest that personal experience and subjective interpretation are *central* to nurse education is a far cry from the narrow definition of 'competence'. Yet, this concept strikes at the heart of the earlier point about assessing counselling skills in a CPN placement. Indeed, how *else* is one to judge interpersonal skills? Burnard highlights the inadequacy of narrowly assessing competence when he suggests a way of combining experiential learning and andragogy: 'Such a combination needs to take into account certain basic principles such as negotiation, the importance of personal experience and the use of self and peer assessment' (Burnard 1989: 302).

It may be useful, or even necessary then, to incorporate self and peer assessment into the process of assessing true nursing competence. True 'nursing competence in the clinical area' calls for more than the ability of student nurses to demonstrate their achievement of certain competences – even if these bear the seal of approval of no less a body than the UKCC. It is not enough to concern ourselves with outcomes. Excellence is not achieved by reducing the art of nursing down to a list of 'psychomotor competencies' (Bowles 1995) or 'particular activities performed to a prescribed standard' (ENB 1988). The clinical area – particularly in mental health nursing – is no longer the controlled, medicalised atmosphere of the ward or clinic but is often likely to be the patient's own home with pets and television, families, door bells and telephones ringing. Working in such an environment, the nurse cannot ignore that the patient is also a person – a fact more easily overlooked when the hospitalised patient is stripped of clothes and possessions, and isolated from his family and friends in a bed surrounded by medical technology. In the latter – the more traditional clinical area – assessment may be easier to control and measure 'scientifically'. The CPN's clinical area is less easily controlled since, in a sense, it is not so much the nurse's clinical area as the patient's.

Drawing on Cook (1991), Milligan asserts that:

> educational methods can be directed at meeting the needs of the educator rather than the needs of the student. The same has been argued for practice where the needs of the nurse and the institution can be met at the expense of the patient.
>
> (Milligan 1995: 26)

If nursing is to be patient-centred, then nurse education needs to be learner-centred. As has been said above, one of the benefits of mentorship is that – all mentors being nurses – a system is in place to ensure that the needs of the learner nurse do not usurp the needs of the patient.

If 'person-centredness' is good for both the art of nursing and the art of teaching, then the same should hold for the art of assessing. At the centre of the assessment process should be, not the assessor with his assessment tools and performance criteria, nor the UKCC with their competences, but the student nurse. Merchant criticises reductionist and misdirected methods of assessment when she writes: 'nurse learners are adult and will be expected to assume professional responsibility and maintain safe standards of practice. They, therefore, need to learn to judge their own performance and that of others' (Merchant 1989: 311). This echoes Burnard's advocacy of self and peer assessment (Burnard 1989). So, good practice in assessing involves being student-centred, as far as this is possible without ceasing to be patient-centred, and should involve a degree of self and peer assessment.

Merchant (after Boydell 1976) notes that 'personal growth (that is, self actualisation) can be seen as professional competence, but this is the very type of learning which is not assessed by using traditional methods' (Merchant 1989). Some might dispute that personal growth (or the ultimate goal of this in Maslovian terms, i.e. self-actualisation) is tantamount to professional competence. Nevertheless, Burnard reminds us that the 1982 syllabus of psychiatric nurse training (ENB 1982) 'was formulated . . . by people who had a considerable interest in humanistic psychology' and that 'many aspects of the syllabus reflect the humanistic approach' (Burnard 1989: 301). I myself am a product of this training and, as such, tend to see competence in psychiatric nursing as equivalent to self-awareness, if not self-actualisation.

In the light of all this, a rejection of the UKCC's narrow definition of competency is inevitable, since it represents a rejection of education as process and, ultimately, nursing as a human activity requiring personal growth. The model is reductionist and behavioural, rather than humanistic and self-actualising. Milligan insists that:

> education cannot be separated out from the wider socio-political climate . . . we must be politically aware and active in our defence of educational methods that we find useful and appropriate, yet are

politically unfashionable or perhaps too challenging, in the wider socio-
political context.

(Milligan 1995: 27)

It was a project funded by the ENB that may have led to the rehabilitation
of 'politically unfashionable' ideas about assessing. The ENB, which, in 1988,
seemed to take such a reductionist approach to the question of competence,
by 1991 had commissioned a wide-ranging study of *The Assessment of
Competencies in Nursing and Midwifery Education and Training* (known as the
'ACE Project'). By 1994, the qualitative research of the ACE Project had
broadened the debate, arguing for 'the conceptualisation of competence as
not a "thing", not an "outcome", but rather a multifaceted process' (Phillips
et al. 1994).

The ACE Project called for the integration of assessment and learning
through structured dialogue, involving students, mentors and link-tutors. It
promoted the ideas of reflective practice, dialogue and partnership. 'What is
required is the knowing subject as a reflective practitioner within a community of reflective practitioners each engaged in critique to improve practice'
(ibid.). It remains to be seen how far the recommendations of the ACE
Project will become part of our nursing culture. What is clear is that the
political climate has begun to change and, as practitioners, mentors and
assessors, we can begin to change things.

In practical terms this means maintaining and promoting our own awareness of ourselves and others within the assessment process. It means focusing
on the process of assessment, as we focus on the processes of learning and of
nursing, rather than allowing ourselves to be obsessed with the outcomes of
these processes. It means opening ourselves up to self-assessment and peer-
assessment, in a negotiated way, so that assessors are not merely gate-keepers
to the profession but truly competent practitioners.

5 Risky business
Risk-taking and safe practice

Reflection

Sometimes in the afternoon they show re-runs of creaky old films and television series. Being of an age where nostalgia is as important as the cutting edge, I sometimes set the video recorder to tape these so that, in our harmless way, we can enjoy them in the evening. Interspersing these broadcasts are frequent advertisements urging people to make a claim for compensation in the case of an accident.

It used to be said that 'accidents will happen' and that, by their nature, they are an inevitable part of life. However, people are now encouraged to believe that someone must be responsible, or negligent, that these things do not 'just happen' and, therefore, somebody must be held accountable, brought to book, made to pay. 'Victims' of accidents are led to believe that they can make money from their misfortune. There is no longer such a thing as 'hard luck'. Tripping on pavements, if we are to believe the advertisements, can lead to big pay-outs. I do not mean here to belittle physical or psychological trauma caused by personal or community disasters but, in everyday life, a little philosophical fatalism might actually be more healthy.

What is called for is a balance between personal and societal responsibility for health and safety. It seems, though, that the public is growing less and less tolerant of any risk of harm and this threatens to paralyse nursing practice with a sense of defensiveness in place of openness and willingness to take chances.

When nurses mention 'risk' nowadays it is usually in the context of 'risk management' or 'risk assessment'. An entire industry has built up supporting mental health workers' need to be seen to be competent in assessing and managing risk. This is fine, as far as it goes. To take one example, if we were to consult *Learning Materials in Mental Health* (Bagley 1996) we would find a helpful checklist of risk factors that indicate increased potential for harm to self and to others. Let us then juxtapose this information with a given patient – for example, a woman with psychotic depression. Using the criteria, we could extrapolate that the patient – being in the older age range, female, divorced, retired and living alone – is at a higher risk of self-harm, and represents a lower risk of harming others (ibid.). Such 'facts' can then influence our practice. We may be reassured that this patient poses less of a threat to others (including ourselves) and we may decide to monitor her more closely for signs of suicidal ideation.

Although it would not stand up in court, so to speak, many skilled CPNs would have already been aware of these 'facts' without having to consult any 'learning materials' on risk assessment, without consciously using this set of indicators or any other particular risk assessment tool. Whether such a tool would reduce the likelihood of the patient harming herself is debatable because, under pressure to take new referrals on to their caseloads, many CPNs would discharge the patient if she were judged to be no longer depressed or psychotic. Awareness of the risk factors could, however, help to inform how we (and the other professionals involved) might manage her care and treatment. For example, the prescription of a Selective Serotonin Reuptake Inhibitor (SSRI) antidepressant in place of a tricyclic would be a sensible measure that would reduce the risk of harm were the patient to take an overdose.

I remain to be convinced that protocols and procedures for assessing and managing risk are preferable to 'clinical judgement' or even 'intuition'. This may not be a safe or politically correct position to maintain in these times of evidence-based practice but it may be less dehumanising for workers and for patients if we use our therapeutic relationships, our knowledge and our skills to promote positive risk-taking on all sides, rather than to try to circumscribe people's lives with checklists and documentation.

When I wrote 'Risk-taking: a nurse's duty' in 1991, I had barely heard of the concept of 'risk management'. Perhaps I was aware of it as a dim noise in the background. I was feeling rebellious and wanted to turn things on their head in order to provoke thought. I suppose I was irritated with the nursing profession for its tendency to 'err on the side of caution'.

I am conscious that the references to the UKCC documents are a little dated now and might have been superseded by revisions in the Code of Conduct. Therefore, I checked with the UKCC and was surprised to hear from them that the dichotomy I highlighted in my article (i.e. the tension between 'safeguarding' and 'promoting well-being) remains in more recent versions of their advice to nurses. I was not at all surprised to learn that the UKCC, quite rightly, had also issued its own guidance on the matter of 'Risk Assessment and Risk Management'.

Risk-taking: a nurse's duty

A risk can be defined as 'a factor, element, or course involving uncertain danger' or as 'a hazard, a chance of bad consequences' (Reader's Digest 1987: 1321; OUP 1982). Knowing this, our gut reaction to the question 'should nurses take risks?' is likely to be a resounding 'no', on the grounds of safety first. Yet, might there be situations where safety should take a back seat?

No doubt many of us place a high value on the right to take risks in our own lives. Nursing may not be noted for being a particularly dangerous profession. Nevertheless, if we, as individuals, value the right to take risks, should we not advocate our patients' right to take risks too?

According to Carson (1990), 'there is a dignity and individuality in being able and allowed to take risks'. By extension, he adds, 'although risks may be frightening and worrying, risk-taking can be the essence of professional responsibility' (Carson 1990: 83).

It is perhaps significant that few nurses have taken the risk of writing on this subject. We may be reassured or humiliated as a profession to learn that the author of the article quoted above is a lecturer in law. Why, then, are nurses reluctant to commit themselves to advocating risk-taking?

I would suggest it has a lot to do with the *UKCC Code of Professional Conduct* and with the issue of accountability. The opening paragraph of the Code states unequivocally: 'Each registered nurse shall act . . . *above all to safeguard* the interests of individual patients' (UKCC 1984) (my italics). The use of the word *safeguard*, defined by the dictionary as 'keeping safe or secure from danger' (Reader's Digest 1987: 1346), would seem to preclude nurses from risk-taking. Indeed, it almost evokes images of keeping our patients in glass cases and under armed guard. Is this really the prime role of the nurse?

Clause one of the Code mercifully elaborates on this. Here, the nurse is required to 'act always in such a way as to promote and safeguard the well being and interests of patients' (UKCC 1984). It could be argued that promoting patients' interests and safeguarding their well-being are two very different things. As Table 5.1 illustrates, while safeguarding might be seen as preserving a status quo, promoting implies a process of active furthering. If taking risks can promote a patient's well-being, then under the Code of Conduct the nurse might be expected to take risks.

Table 5.1 The dichotomy of 'safeguarding' and 'promoting' well-being

Safeguarding	Promoting
'Keeping safe or secure from danger . . . protecting'	'Contributing to the process or growth of (the patient), furthering'
Static	Dynamic
Negative	Positive
Reactive	Active
Conservative	Innovative

Carson highlights the need to distinguish between a gamble, a risk and a dilemma. A gamble is entirely optional. You may gain something or lose something. Even in losing, a gamble may be pleasurable but it is not necessarily all that therapeutic. A dilemma often involves having to act. Sooner or later, doing nothing will prove harmful. A genuine risk, then, is where a conscious decision is taken 'to achieve specific goals, in the light of possible harm occurring' (Carson 1990: 85). For example, a patient being treated for schizophrenia with a long-acting depot injection may ask for the dosage of his or her medication to be reduced. In so doing, the patient suffers far less from side-effects and feels one day able to completely discontinue the medication.

The specific goal of reducing the side-effects of the medication is a worthy one. The possible harm is that, by reducing the medication, the patient may suffer an acute recurrence of the illness.

Other benefits of the above might be manifold. The reduced frequency of visits by the CPN allows for greater numbers of patients to be seen. Patients may regard themselves as less 'ill' because they find they can survive on less medication, and so on. Often, when we list all the possible benefits of a risk, it can seem irresponsible *not* to take that risk. One might almost say there is a 'duty' to take it.

In Table 5.2, Carson's 13-point framework for risk-taking is laid out. Of particular interest are points eleven and twelve. It is essential under the Code of Conduct that patients should give their informed consent. Moreover, by involving patients, it ceases to be the nurse alone who takes the risk. Patients take the risk for themselves. Any nurse advocating a patient-centred approach has to recognise the importance of self-determinism in risk-taking, as a means to personal growth and change.

Table 5.2 A risk-taking assessment strategy (adapted from Carson (1990))

1. Is the proposed action a gamble, a risk or a dilemma?
2. List all the possible benefits, for the patient, of acting.
3. List all the possible benefits for other people.
4. How likely are these to occur?
5. Manipulate the risk by taking steps to make the benefits more likely to occur.
6. List all the possible kinds of harm, to the patient, of acting.
7. List all the possible kinds of harm to other people.
8. How likely are these to occur?
9. Manipulate the risk by taking steps to reduce the likelihood of harm occurring.
10. List 'duties to risk'.
11. Obtain the patient's informed consent.
12. Obtain the informed consent of colleagues.
13. Assess whether the 'risk' should be taken.

There are two further factors that may seem to stand in the way of risk-taking. These are Clauses Six and Seven of Section H of the Summary of the UKCC policy document, *Exercising Accountability* (UKCC 1989). Clause Six states that 'public trust and confidence in the profession is dependent on its practitioners being seen to exercise their accountability responsibly' (ibid.). Clause Seven says, 'each registered nurse must be able to justify any action or decision not to act taken in the course of her professional practice' (ibid.).

In the face of all this, dare we take the risk of risk-taking? Ironically, the same document on accountability also contains the two elements that make risk-taking safer and more justifiable. *Exercising Accountability* stresses the importance of advocacy on behalf of patients.

As we have said, if we value our own right to take risks, we should uphold that right for patients. Second, the document emphasises the importance of collaboration and co-operation in care with other health care professionals. This is, happily, point twelve of Carson's framework. What this amounts to is making sure that the decision to take a risk is not solely your decision. It is paramount that the decision to take a risk is a multi-disciplinary team decision.

If nothing else, perhaps all this highlights the importance of taking risks and the importance of minimising the dangers. What seems to be a contradiction in our professional code is, on reflection, a dichotomy that brings into focus two stances in nursing – whether to safeguard or promote well-being. While we go on safeguarding our patients' well-being, we may be missing the chance to promote it.

Reflection

By the end of the 1990s clinical supervision may not have been such a new idea. Nevertheless, when I wrote my short article 'Some thoughts on clinical supervision' it seemed to me I was still in a minority of nurses who received supervision in practice. I had been lucky enough to have a team leader who felt strongly about it and was wise enough to insist on every member of the CPN team receiving regular, formal supervision from a colleague of their choice. This elegantly made it a requirement while empowering each CPN to exercise some freedom in their choice of supervisor.

Since writing 'Some thoughts on clinical supervision' I have become involved in supervision in a different way. After training in Behavioural Family Therapy (BFT), and subsequently training as a BFT Trainer, I have been responsible for providing group supervision, focusing specifically on family work to those people whom I have helped to train. I have also had the privilege of receiving such supervision as part of the regional programme in family interventions described in Chapter 10. This has enabled me to compare individual supervision with group supervision and to appreciate even more the support and creativity of family interventions practitioners from a range of disciplines.

Just as training can benefit from being provided in a multi-disciplinary way, so can supervision. As I suggested in Chapter 3, psychiatric nurses have more in common with mental health workers from other disciplines, than they do with other nurses. It is salutary for CPNs to share their ideas about their own practice with other mental health professionals. For example, one psychologist said to me, 'If CPNs are not comfortable doing something structured and purposeful with patients, what exactly do they normally do?' I hope that this book will give people a good overview of what it is that CPNs do, although we may not always be terribly clear about this ourselves.

I think there is a place for CPNs to scrutinise what we do and to compare our approaches with those of other disciplines. (Family therapy group supervision provides excellent opportunities for this.) The ideal is probably that CPNs should have some multi-disciplinary training and supervision, and some training and supervision purely within their own discipline. Perhaps by comparing notes between individual CPN-to-CPN supervision and multi-disciplinary group supervision, CPNs will become clearer about what we do, and how and why we do it.

Some thoughts on clinical supervision

The Department of Health, the ENB, the UKCC, all say we should be doing it. Perhaps even your own nurse manager is urging you to have clinical supervision. Despite this, or possibly because of it, you may be one of the many nurses who remain suspicious of the idea.

In recent years, clinical supervision in nursing has been promoted by an onslaught of reports from various organisations. But it is hardly a new idea, as Farrington (1998) points out. Clinical supervision has been

> a feature of professional activity for people working in counselling and psychotherapy for at least twenty years, including psychiatric and mental health nurses . . . although its introduction to date into general nursing and into many areas of mental health nursing appears piecemeal and infrequent.
>
> (Farrington 1998: 19)

For those who remain sceptical, or even perhaps blissfully unaware of what is involved, I thought it might be helpful to share my own experience of clinical supervision. I have been receiving supervision on a fortnightly basis since I became a CPN nearly eight years ago. At the start, I was looking for guidance about whether I was 'CPNing' properly. Should I try to keep this patient out of hospital, should I push for his admission, did I need to arrange for him to see a consultant or would it be enough for me to have a chat about him with his GP? My supervisor had been a CPN for a few years more than me and seemed very much like a 'mentor'; an experienced, or even 'expert', CPN who could help me to make these decisions for myself.

Much fun or tedious academic argument, depending on your viewpoint, is to be had trying to distinguish between mentorship, preceptorship and clinical supervision. The boundaries between these concepts seem to blur.

My understanding is that mentorship is something learners receive, whereas preceptorship is something trained nurses receive when they find themselves in a new role or clinical area. In contrast to mentorship and preceptorship, which should be provided at different stages of our professional development, supervision is something that should be available continuously throughout our nursing career. I suspect even our governing bodies get confused about the precise definitions.

At the beginning of my career in community psychiatric nursing, supervision seemed to be part of a process of developing expertise and, I am glad to say, it continues to fulfil this function. As a result of these years of receiving supervision, though, I have developed a greater ability to supervise myself and to reflect upon the sort of questions I would previously have needed to 'check' with my supervisor. It gives me confidence in my own decision-making and is a fundamental element of 'reflective practice', another factor that our governing bodies ask us – quite rightly – to take into account.

Alongside receiving my own supervision, I have been approached by several others to offer supervision to them. I find this very enriching because colleagues tell me the story of their day-to-day clinical dilemmas, anxieties and achievements from different perspectives. I supervise one CPN colleague from the 'elderly' team and one from the 'adult' team. I also act as clinical supervisor to two colleagues from HomeStart (a non-statutory organisation that provides volunteers to support young families under stress – discussed more fully in Chapter 6).

All this giving and receiving supervision typically takes up six hours a month. Some managers may question this time commitment but I consider it time well spent in terms of the mutual learning that takes place, the team-building, the reduction of workplace stress and the increased efficiency of reflective, well-thought-out casework. In other words, patients ultimately benefit from a higher-quality service.

There are many models of clinical supervision but I believe in the school of thought that says supervision should be highly challenging at the same time as being highly supportive. In this way, it avoids being self-congratulatory or smug.

The supervision I have received has been invaluable, not only in deciding how best to work with patients but also in working out how I feel about colleagues and myself, and what I do and do not want to be doing in my work. It has helped me feel better about my job and has helped me to decide *not* to look for another one.

Supervision is a powerful force for recruitment and retention, and any public-service employer that fails to offer it is short-changing its workers, risking losing employees and dooming its patients and clients to a mediocre service. If you were one of those nurses who doubted its usefulness, why go on waiting for your managers to impose clinical supervision upon you? Seek them out and ask why you have not been offered it already.

6   If you're happy and you know it
Promoting positive mental health

Reflection

I wonder who first used the phrase 'crazy mixed-up kids'? It conjures up images of the older generation failing to understand the turmoil of youth. The generation gap, of course, is two-sided. Young people do their own thing, older people fail to understand it. In some ways, this is the way of the world. It is the force that propels young people into adulthood, encouraging them to leave home and become independent, and also the force that encourages older people to put down roots and 'stay put'. This struggle is portrayed vividly in popular culture. In films and musicals and pop songs from *Fiddler on the Roof* to Cat Stevens' *Father and Son*. Children, as they become teenagers, are expected to become a little 'crazy' and 'mixed-up', which makes it difficult to know whether this change is a sign of mental health or mental illness.

Psychiatric nurse training has traditionally focused on mental illness in adults and the idea that children can be mentally unwell is a relatively recent concept. Nurses specialising in 'children and adolescents' are still few in number and organisations (like YoungMinds) concerned with the mental health of children are only now gathering momentum.

Working with families (rather than solely with individual adults) brings generic CPNs into contact with children and young people. Being a parent (or an aunt or uncle) may give you a few clues on how to work with children but, when so much professional time is spent with adults, it can be a disorientating experience. We cannot afford to neglect the mental health of children and young people, even if we are employed primarily to work with adults. If we are serious about 'health promotion' and 'early intervention' (what might be called '*really* early intervention') it is essential that we create opportunities to work with the younger age group, be this through careers guidance or health promotion activities with schools (such as those described in the articles 'What's it worth?' and 'Second that emotion'), or through family interventions (as described in Chapter 10).

Initiatives, like World Mental Health Day and, more recently, the National Service Framework for Mental Health, have given a renewed legitimacy to CPNs' involvement in mental health promotion. Standard One of the

National Service Framework, for instance, states that health and social services should 'promote mental health for all, working with individuals and communities' (Department of Health 2000). We can assume children are included in the phrase 'working with individuals and communities', since The Children Act 1989 reminds us that all children should be treated as individuals and with equal concern.

It should not require legislation to remind CPNs that all children should be treated as individuals or that the welfare of the child is paramount. It ought to be obvious. Perhaps, in becoming adults, we learn to become dismissive of the tremendous power and influence we have over children's development. This consequence can be tragic – as described in 'What's it worth?' – or tragi-comic. Garrison Keillor (in *Lake Wobegon Days*) describes the lasting impact parents' injunctions can have on our lives, whether we comply or rebel against these:

> Because you always went to bed at ten, I stayed up half the night chain-smoking (you were opposed to cigarettes), drinking straight gin (you didn't drink), and, given time, might have cut off my arm, it being yet another thing you would never have done.

(Keillor 1986: 269)

What's it worth?

On 8 April 1994, Kurt Cobain, guitarist and singer with the grunge band Nirvana, was found dead. Toxicology reports indicated his blood contained three times the fatal dose of heroin but the cause of death was a self-inflicted gunshot wound to the head.

I was shocked by the news. I had only recently become aware of Nirvana's music, having been given the band's album *In Utero* as a present. Cobain himself described that album as having 'the sound I have been carrying around in my head since the beginning of the band'. It saddened me to think Cobain would produce no more of this extraordinary music.

A month later I was invited to spend the afternoon at a local high school. The object of the exercise was to give teenage boys an insight into the work of a CPN. A group of 15-year-old boys can be something of a shock when you are used to working with adults all day. After a while, though, I was able to draw on some long-forgotten teaching experience and, combining it with a few techniques from group therapy, was able to effect a form of crowd control.

It had been a couple of decades since I was a teenage boy myself, so it took a while to tune into their particular style of communicating. I hope they learnt something about community psychiatric nursing. Hackneyed as it sounds, though, I doubt if they learnt as much from me as I learnt from them.

The students brought with them some interesting myths, surprisingly not so much about male nurses but about mental health. The term 'psycho' was used frequently to denote one suffering from mental illness. It seemed shorthand for 'psychopath' rather than for 'person with a psychotic illness' and the assumption was that my caseload was made up of dangerous and deranged killers.

Most interesting was the idea that mental illness might be 'catching'. Some of the students were wary of contemplating a career in mental health for fear of succumbing to mental illness themselves. But there was also a preoccupation with Kurt Cobain, whose recent suicide had clearly touched a nerve. The students' fascination with suicide was conveyed through black humour and I wondered if this typically male defence would have been dropped had it been a mixed group.

I remember one of the school group asking me, with mock seriousness, 'Could you have stopped Kurt Cobain from killing himself? If he'd had a community nurse visiting him, would that have sorted him out?' Some of them showed a very mature awareness that drug abuse – more likely to be solvents than heroin – could lead to mental illness. Others recognised that mental illness can be caused by grief, separation and abuse. Cobain was a case in point; devastated at the age of eight by his parents' separation, subsequently beaten by his father, he grew up feeling worthless. The working title of *In Utero* was *I Hate Myself and I Want to Die*. It might seem tragic that so many teenagers identify with the music born of these sentiments but it should not surprise us.

At a memorial service, Nirvana's bassist, Krist Novoselic, tried to console fans with this message:

> Let's keep the music with us, we'll always have it, forever. Kurt had an ethic towards his fans which was rooted in a punk rock way of thinking. No band is special, no player royalty. If you've got a guitar and a lot of soul, just bang something out and mean it. You're the superstar.

Cobain did not consider himself a superstar. He made it clear how little he thought of himself in his songs: 'I'm a stain', he sang, 'I'm so ugly', and 'I think I'm dumb'.

People who left their teens behind a few years ago have a responsibility for the mental health of our society. They may think the lesson to be learnt from Kurt Cobain's death is simply 'heroin kills'. That is one lesson to be drawn. Another is that our children and young people need, more than anything, to feel they are worth something. Society needs to allow people to feel their own worth, to be their own superstars. The tragedy is not just that Kurt Cobain fulfilled his wish for the void. It is that he, and so many others, feel it is the only wish they deserve.

Reflection

I have always thought there are two sides to mental health promotion. On the one hand is the idea of promoting positive mental health either in individuals or in the general population. On the other hand is the aspect of promoting a more positive image of mentally ill people in our community. This is closely linked with reducing stigma. Working with non-statutory organisations can provide great opportunities for both of these aspects.

In 'Working with HomeStart' I describe my involvement with an organisation whose links with mental health are not obvious. Many CPNs work closely with organisations like MIND and the National Schizophrenia Fellowship (NSF). These organisations attract workers (some paid, many voluntary) who do excellent work and who often have great knowledge, awareness and skill in the field of mental health. HomeStart's main focus is the welfare of children and families, and not explicitly people with mental health problems. However, given the prevalence of mental health problems in our society, HomeStart inevitably finds itself concerned with mental health.

Because of this difference in focus, HomeStart's workers may be relatively uninformed about mental illness. In many ways, HomeStart volunteers are typical members of the public. They are all parents or grandparents whose knowledge of mental illness is limited to that garnered from the mass media, unless, of course, they have suffered with mental health problems in their own right. It would be surprising, as a cross-section of the public, if a number of volunteers had not suffered with depression and anxiety, and, in fact, many of them have been drawn to the work because of their own experience of postnatal depression.

Training HomeStart volunteers, then, is very different to training mental health workers. I generally find them an experienced and compassionate group of people but they often know very little about major mental illness. For example, they may believe schizophrenia is a 'Jekyll and Hyde' condition. They know what depression is but not necessarily what 'manic-depressive' means. They may believe antidepressants are addictive. They may think 'schizophrenics' are likely to be dangerous. They may not know what the difference is between a psychiatrist and a psychologist. And why should they? All this is typical of what the general public 'knows'. What a wonderful opportunity, then, to put the record straight. To teach these members of the public something more accurate about the nature and treatment of schizophrenia, bi-polar illness and depression.

Of course, there is a limit to what can be conveyed in a brief training session. I try to give volunteers an opportunity to reflect on what they know about mental health and to dispel a few myths. I also try to help them build up a picture of how they fit into a range of helping agencies and how they might help an individual or family access professional help if required. In doing so, I like to think that I am reducing the stigma of mental illness in a few members of the public and providing them with the means to contribute towards the recovery of people with mental health problems.

My training of the volunteers is complemented by the supervision I provide to the scheme's co-ordinators. This helps to ensure that where, for example, there is a difficulty between a volunteer and a family, the co-ordinators have a forum for exploring ways of dealing with this. As described in Chapter 5, supervision seems to have a function, not just of improving the service provided but of making workers feel more comfortable about the difficulties they face in their practice. Thus, through the supervision and support of the co-ordinators, we are all working together to promote the mental health of the volunteers themselves and the families they help.

Working with HomeStart

In 1998, HomeStart celebrated 25 years of voluntary work, supporting young families under stress. Despite this anniversary, many health professionals have little awareness of the organisation. In July of that year the government announced that it would be setting up Sure Start – a new strategy which has much in common with the aims of HomeStart and which equally deserves wider attention. This article seeks to explain more about HomeStart and about the Sure Start initiative, while focusing in particular on one local HomeStart scheme, HomeStart Wyre Forest.

HomeStart UK is a national non-statutory organisation committed to promoting the welfare of families with at least one child under five years. Its volunteers offer regular support, friendship and practical help to families in their own homes, helping to prevent family crisis and breakdown. Volunteers are normally parents themselves (some are even grandparents) who offer their time freely. All HomeStart volunteers undergo an initial preparation course and, with support and ongoing training, they are able to draw on their own parenting experience, their own skills and local knowledge of the resources available to families. Having no official status, they do not represent 'authority', so families find them less threatening than they might find workers from the statutory agencies.

The HomeStart approach is based on home-visiting and supporting parents and their children in whichever ways the family finds most useful. With a caring but realistic attitude, volunteers seek to build on the strengths of the family, sharing time and friendship so that families are able to develop new relationships, ideas and skills. The support offered may be different from, but complementary to, that provided by professionals, such as health visitors, social workers and community nurses. Visiting will continue for as long as the family feels it appropriate. It can last from a few months to a year or more and, of course, families can opt out at any time. The aim is that the family will become empowered through the personal relationship they develop with their volunteer.

Though not normally a crisis-intervention service, volunteers may be able to respond to a crisis in the family once a relationship has been established. *HomeStart's Policy and Practice Guide* describes their aim as being to give support to families 'to prevent difficulties escalating into crises, and crises from developing into family breakdown'.

Volunteers can offer a listening ear, reassurance and practical help with the children. They can give parents a break so that families get the opportunity to meet other parents, or help people to access local resources, keep appointments or renew links with family and friends. This is not to say the volunteer is a free alternative to 'home-helps' or baby-sitters. The intention is to be seen more like a friend of the family, who is willing to give help without being judgemental. Being a parent is, arguably, the most difficult job anyone could be asked to do and most of us take it on without any formal training. The volunteer can be a useful role model – one of HomeStart's favourite phrases is 'parenting skills can be "caught" rather than "taught"'.

The first scheme opened in 1973 in Leicester. There are now over 200 schemes scattered throughout the UK. Each of these is an independent charity, locally managed by a multi-disciplinary management committee. All the schemes are locally funded and employ co-ordinators, responsible for recruiting, training, supporting and supervising volunteers. The local schemes receive training, guidance and support from HomeStart UK.

So, if this is HomeStart what is Sure Start? Sure Start is a government strategy to help children under four and their families. Brian Waller, HomeStart's director, welcomed Sure Start as 'a radical government programme to target help into socially deprived communities across the UK'. Over a period of three years the government is committing more than £500 million to the initiative, planning first to introduce it in England and then to develop it in Scotland, Wales and Northern Ireland. 'Within the Sure Start projects', explained the organisation's director, 'it is hoped that HomeStart schemes will be able to make a substantial contribution, offering the HomeStart service to all families in the related areas.'

In January 1999, the government announced what they described as sixty 'trailblazer' districts in England. I was privileged to meet a few of the original 'trailblazers' of HomeStart long before the New Labour government discovered such schemes were a good idea. While HomeStart UK was celebrating its first 25 years, one local scheme was happy to be celebrating its first two years. HomeStart Wyre Forest serves families in the Worcestershire town of Kidderminster and the surrounding district; the same 'patch' where I work as a CPN. Since its inception, the original co-ordinators, Sheila Lockwood and Ellen Dolphin, worked hard to foster excellent links with our CPN department.

I first became aware of HomeStart through the Community Resources Development Group (CRDG). The CRDG is a local forum of health, social services and non-statutory workers in the field of mental health. Ellen and Sheila invited themselves to come along and speak with the CRDG and this was the beginning of HomeStart Wyre Forest aligning itself with local mental health workers. Those of us in the field of mental health are always being urged to work in a co-operative and collaborative way with other agencies and it was not long before my CPN colleagues and I recognised the crucial role that HomeStart could play alongside us.

First, CPNs were able to refer families with whom we were involved and where there was a family member with mental illness. This is vitally important as, along with our health visitor colleagues, we recognise the high incidence of post-natal depression in a locality that has no specialist in-patient 'mother and baby' facilities. Apart from depression, it is not uncommon for people with major mental illnesses, such as schizophrenia and manic depression, to have young children, and collaborative work between mental health workers and HomeStart has been very fruitful.

Second, there is an increasing emphasis on mental health promotion. There are two aspects to this. On the one hand, it includes promoting positive mental health in the general population. On the other hand, it is also about promoting a more positive image of mentally ill people in our community. CPN links with HomeStart facilitate both of these aims, to the benefit of those we call our clients or patients and the community as a whole.

Third, liaison between CPNs and HomeStart in the form of training, formal supervision, support and sharing of resources, has been an enriching experience for everyone involved. This pooling of resources has included very practical things like the co-ordinators allowing CPNs to use the local scheme's rooms from time to time for group work. I have been involved in the training of volunteers and in supervising the co-ordinators (see Chapter 5) and I have always found this a breath of 'fresh air', as HomeStart workers often have a very different perspective to those of us who work for the health service.

One of the remarkable things about the group is the way in which everyone connected with it is encouraged to develop their potential more fully. In this spirit, one of the original co-ordinators left to pursue a career as a psychologist. The other half of the original partnership is still co-ordinating HomeStart Wyre Forest while, at the same time, training to become a social worker. The original secretary has left to start her own business and, in doing so, created a vacancy that was filled by one of the original volunteers, while another former volunteer has taken up a post of co-ordinator.

HomeStart Wyre Forest is not in a 'trailblazer district', as identified by the Sure Start initiative. Despite this, the local group goes on to achieve a great deal and, as Sure Start expands, it is hoped more resources will be available to support and extend its work.

It is said that 'the whole is greater than the sum of its parts' and this is well illustrated by the special relationship that has grown up between the HomeStart co-ordinators, the volunteers, the CPN department and our colleagues in health and social services. Together, we have been able to achieve far more than we could have done as separate agencies. Up and down the country, schemes like HomeStart Wyre Forest, with the competence and confidence of their co-ordinators and volunteers, are enhancing the mental health of the community and reducing the stress felt by young families.

Reflection

After the publication of my article 'Second that emotion' in 1999, my manager requested 'a quick word' with me. He was delighted that I had had something published but was rather perturbed by the closing paragraph. He felt that the article seemed to be implying that management had been unsupportive of my contribution towards World Mental Health Day. I was rather wrong-footed because I had not seen the published article which, the editor of *Nursing Times* had warned me, had needed a severe cutting down to size to fit the page.

It seems it had lost some of my diplomacy in the editing process and so I had to make up a swift apologia to make my manager feel better. Well, first, I had a different manager at the time of writing. Secondly, *Nursing Times* had altered the sense of what I was saying through their ruthless editing. Thirdly, I was *not* saying management had been unsupportive, just that they had not discussed it a great deal with me. Fourthly, this was probably my own fault because the whole thing was a bit of an experiment, I had been uncertain how it would go and, therefore, had deliberately kept it low-profile (this last point was actually included in the published article).

There are lessons to be learnt here. Although I am keen to encourage nurses to write and get their writing published (see Chapter 4), this should carry with it a word of caution. The reactions of managers and colleagues when they read your published work can vary from approval to paranoia. The old saying 'publish and be damned!' cannot be espoused too enthusiastically if you wish to enjoy a convivial working environment.

The second lesson to be learnt is that sometimes it may be better to publicise your plans (however experimental they might be) before carrying them out. This is difficult as you run the risk of making a fool of yourself twice (once at the planning stage and once when it fails in practice!). There is a risk that, if your ideas are too innovative, others will put obstacles in your way. On the other hand, occasionally managers and colleagues can come up with helpful suggestions of which you (working away at an idea by yourself) would never have dreamt.

Whatever managers, colleagues or participants feel, before or after the event, it is always helpful to have some external evaluation of your efforts. The Health Education Authority provided a useful summary of key findings from World Mental Health Day in 1997 and this stressed the importance of systematic and clear-sighted evaluation of the Day's activities. This is certainly something that was lacking from the activity I carried out. I used no formal means for assessing the effectiveness of what I did and I relied purely on informally asking teachers for feedback. Having some form of formal evaluation would, of course, have helped to demonstrate the effectiveness of my work, not only to the school and the community but also to my managers. This would have provided an objective framework for deciding on the value of similar activities in the future.

It seems likely that the National Service Framework, while 'giving permission', as it were, for CPNs to engage in health promotion activities, will also require these activities to be 'evidence-based'. We, therefore, need to learn what types of activities are effective and hope that, in being guided by evidence, we do not lose our sense of innovation and our spirit of adventure.

Second that emotion

World Mental Health Day (10 October) involves thousands of communities across the globe in raising awareness of mental health needs. In 1997, I decided to celebrate this day by combining my roles as CPN and school governor. I spent the day at my son's school, reaching out to the most impressionable members of the local community with a message of positive mental health.

Parent governors who want a quiet life traditionally offer to pop in and listen to a few children reading. I, being foolish and new to the role, and being a CPN in the run-up to World Mental Health Day, decided here was an opportunity to kill two birds with one stone.

One of the teachers had already suggested that I should bring my guitar in to entertain the children. I was used to using music-making as a means of promoting mental health through my work with the Music Workshop Project (see Chapter 8). It was natural, then, for me to decide to combine music and mental health in my sessions with the children.

I chose, as the central focus for my session, a song that all the children recognised – *If you're happy and you know it clap your hands* – to explore how music can express different moods. I demonstrated this by playing the song quickly, brightly, loudly and in the major key (which the children recognised as 'happy') and then repeating the song slowly, sombrely and quietly in the minor ('sad') key. This was followed by a discussion about why we associate different tempos, different textures of sound, different levels of volume and different musical 'modes' (major and minor) with different moods. I had to adjust the language I used to the vocabulary, comprehension and emotional understanding of the different groups of children (who were all between the ages of five and nine).

The children enjoyed singing and clapping along, and also simply listening to a live musical performance, which, for many of them, is a rare experience. One of the teachers introduced an interesting idea – that she enjoyed the 'sad' version more than the 'happy' one. This led on to a surprisingly sophisticated discussion about how music does not always match our moods, how 'sad' music can lift the spirits while 'happy' music can sometimes heighten our awareness that we are not feeling happy.

Another interesting point arising from this was how quickly our moods can change and how it sometimes does not take much to change the way we feel. I illustrated this by showing how the difference between major and minor – 'happy' and 'sad' – is just one slight movement of one finger on the guitar, one fret, one semitone. Again, no knowledge of musical theory is necessary to see and hear this difference. In the words (and the music) of the old Cole Porter song: 'How strange the change from major to minor, every time we say goodbye'.

As well as using music as a starting point for discussion, I also used a set of activity sheets that had been specially produced by the Health Education Authority as a resource for World Mental Health Day. I supplied these to the head teacher in advance of my visit and was delighted to learn that several classes had been using them prior to my visit. The activity sheets, which some of the younger children liked to colour in, used cartoon pictures to depict situations and encouraged the children to imagine, for example, how a spaceman from Mars might feel when his space craft has crash-landed in their back garden. What could you do to make him feel better?

One of the most thought-provoking activity sheets showed a series of doors leading to the angry room, the fun room, the happy room, the sad room and the scary room. It showed a child trying to decide what might be behind each of these doors. The fun room was generally considered to contain ice cream and computer games. The happy room contained friends, while the sad room was a room with no toys and no friends with which to play. The children recognised that boredom and loneliness could lead to sadness. The scary room and the angry room were felt to contain parents having arguments.

Another activity sheet showed parents apparently having a stand-up argument while a hapless child tried to watch television. The teacher and I posed the questions, not only 'How would you feel?' but 'What could you do about it?' One child cried out: 'Lock 'em in!'

The activity sheets touched on bullying and ostracism, on getting bad marks from the teacher, on feeling an outsider at school. I tried to promote the empathic imagination of the children by asking them to look at each of these scenarios from the differing points of view of different characters. How would they feel if they had just smashed a neighbour's window with their football and, on the other hand, how might the neighbour feel?

The feedback from the school was very positive and provided the opportunity for spreading the messages of World Mental Health Day to the parents and the wider community, through the session itself, through out-of-school work and discussion which it triggered off. The event was even mentioned in the *Governors' Report to Parents*. I was also heartened to have direct feedback from parents who told me their children had proudly taken home their worksheets and that this had led to further discussion in the home between parents and children about mental health issues. My musical efforts had also inspired some children to express an interest in learning to play a musical instrument!

Feedback from my own managers was less evident but this was partly because I had not made my activities well known at work. Although our CPN department has a policy of promoting positive mental health, I did not feel over-confident about how the session would go and so I had kept my plans deliberately low-profile. Minutes before I left for the school, on the actual morning of World Mental Health Day, I received a message from my managers: 'Does anybody know if anybody's doing anything about World Mental Health Day?' I replied that I was but I could not stop to discuss it! I wondered whether they would be pleased that I was getting involved in proactively promoting positive mental health or whether they would bemoan the fact that I was allowing myself to be distracted from my face-to-face work with mentally ill people. I gather that they were pleased that, in the end, somebody had done something to mark the event.

7   Totally atypical taste

Coming to terms with newer treatments

Reflection

Advertisements for more senior psychiatric nursing jobs sometimes ask for 'a relevant degree'. If you ask what subjects of degree are considered relevant (as I have occasionally) you will be told psychology or sociology. My degree (in English and French) has never been considered 'relevant'. It has even been the subject of amused puzzlement at a few job interviews I have endured, but – far from writing off four years of my life as an irrelevant prelude to my nursing career – I have always tried to 'positively re-frame' my degree as one infinitely relevant to psychiatric nursing. Rather in the spirit of the Polish psychologist, who admitted, 'We psychologists are only the plumbers of the psyche. It is the novelists and playwrights who are the poets of human inter-action' (O'Brien and Houston 2000: 76).

For one thing, studying language and literature leads to a sensitivity towards meaning and an ability to move from the metaphorical to the literal. This is extremely useful when communicating with people with psychosis, as is the skill of speaking, reading, writing and listening in a different language (which, of course, involves ultimately *thinking* in a different language). What better ways of developing empathic communication and the ability to advocate on one another's behalf, than by learning to think and express oneself with terms of reference from outside one's natural culture, and to study the arts of interpreting and translation?

When I stumbled across neuro-linguistic programming (NLP), it intrigued me because of this interplay between linguistics and psychology. I thought, whether it worked or not, that it was an entertaining idea. I was working weekends in a nursing home, to make up a shortfall in income, having just given up nights for days. I found myself working alongside a character who had become self-employed in order to combine agency nursing with a career as a hypno-therapist. It was he who told me about NLP. I suppose I have always seen it as an 'alternative' form of psychotherapy or counselling, with not much in the way of an 'evidence-base'.

'Evidence-base' or not, like Transactional Analysis, NLP has a surprising hold over psychiatric nurses. Training courses appear from time to time, lecturers in nursing will provide sessions on it for their students, the nursing press will publish the occasional article about it. In 1993, *Nursing Times* rejected 'Representational systems in counselling' because they had recently published another article on NLP. *Nursing Standard* published it, with the introductory words: 'the theories of NLP are becoming more popular in shaping the approaches of nurses to counselling'.

When writing this section on 'atypical' treatments, it occurred to me that the subject goes beyond 'typical' and 'atypical' drugs. NLP is, as it were, an 'atypical' psychological intervention. You may wish to dismiss it as an intervention with little evidence to support its use, in which case, you can read the article as pure entertainment. If you think there might be something useful in it, then I hope you will find it a clear exposition of one aspect of NLP. The article grew out of a workshop that I did with some CPN colleagues. I have taken this opportunity to alter the ludicrous and fictitious name of 'Dr O Dittrey' on the suggestion of one of the participants in the workshop, who felt it should be, not an initial and surname, but the quasi-Irish-sounding (but no less absurd) 'Dr O'Dittrey'.

Representational systems in counselling

Neuro-linguistic programming (NLP) is becoming increasingly popular as a theory in the areas of learning and communication. It was originally developed by two Americans, Bandler and Grinder, drawing on theory from linguistics, neurophysiology and other fields. Their ideas and observations were set out in the seminal NLP text, *Frogs Into Princes* (Bandler and Grinder 1979). Parts of the theory seem particularly adaptable to counselling and those with an eclectic approach might find it a helpful addition to their therapeutic 'toolkit'.

I first read about NLP's concept of 'representational systems' in *Basic Personal Counselling*, a highly recommended book by the Australian psychologist David Geldard (1989). The theory is that we record, store and recall experiences and thoughts in three sensory modalities – the auditory, visual and kinesthetic (sic). Clearly, auditory relates to hearing and visual to sight. The less familiar term 'kinesthetic' relates to the sense of bodily position, presence or movement, which results from the stimulation of sensory nerve endings in muscles, tendons and joints.

Each individual has a favoured sense, which, in NLP, is called his or her 'primary representational system'. A person's primary representational system is that sensory modality which is used predominantly when accessing (taking in) or processing (making sense of) information.

O'Connor and Seymour (1990) point out how different kinds of psychotherapy show a representational system bias. For instance, bodywork therapies are primarily kinesthetic while psychoanalysis, with its emphasis on speaking and listening, is predominantly verbal and auditory. Art therapy is visually based but so, in a less obvious way, is Jungian symbolism.

According to NLP theory, a client's representational system can be determined by observing his or her speech pattern and voice tones, breathing pattern, gross hand movements and 'preferred predicates'. A good account of these more bizarre-sounding aspects of NLP is given in Wilson and Kneisl (1988) but what interests us now is the concept of 'preferred predicates'. A predicate is a verb, adjective or adverb in a sentence that tells us something about the subject. The examples given below will make clear how such a concept can be applied to NLP.

Since learning of representational systems, I have applied the theory in counselling situations where it has seemed particularly difficult to establish rapport. Where clients have appeared hostile, suspicious, or perhaps just not quite on the same wavelength, I have found it worthwhile consciously noting the representational system within which they tend to operate. It seems that in cases where I have deliberately tried to match with the client's primary representational system, rapport has improved. This very subjective observation would seem to support O'Connor and Seymour's prescription: 'To create rapport, match predicates with the other person. You will be speaking their language, and presenting ideas in just the way they think about them' (O'Connor and Seymour 1990).

All this is perhaps not as magical as it would seem. To match a person's style of verbalising thoughts and emotions is simply to demonstrate a level of empathy. What is different is the deliberate analysis of the client's speech, so that the primary representational system can be discovered and then used by the counsellor.

If the distinction between visual, auditory and kinesthetic systems is still unclear, the following illustration may be helpful. This material can easily be adapted for use in role-play situations, so that you can explore the representational systems and familiarise yourself with the concept.

As a first illustration, let us take Mr Ken S Tettik – a depressed client whose primary representational system is *kinesthetic*. The following description is written using kinesthetic predicates to give a 'feel' of the kinesthetic representational system.

> Since being made redundant six weeks ago, Mr Tettik has been feeling increasingly depressed. He feels irritable and cannot bear to stay indoors. He is beginning to feel out of touch with reality. At night he has unpleasant sensations of being cornered by his situation. In the mornings he wakes up feeling 'heavy'. He feels he is a burden to his family.

Now, imagine that Mr Tettik goes to his GP who refers him to the CPN team. The GP that Mr Tettik sees is one whose primary representational system is visual – one Dr V Zyewell! Dr V Zyewell's letter to the CPNs might look something like this:

Letter from Dr V Zyewell re Mr Ken S Tettik

Thank you for agreeing to see this gentleman. At first sight, it seems to be a simple case of reactive depression. But having taken a closer look at his family history, it becomes clear that he has always looked on the dark side of things. At present, he can see no way out of his depression. He is looking forward to seeing you, however, and I regard this as a good sign. It seems he was made redundant six weeks ago. He says he finds it difficult staring at the same four walls every day. His view of reality is becoming somewhat distorted. He is also neglecting his appearance, which hardly helps his self-image at the moment.

The referral letter from Dr Zyewell is framed in the visual representational system. Look at it again, but this time with all the visual representational references highlighted:

Thank you for agreeing to *see* this gentleman. *At first sight*, it *seems* to be a simple case of reactive depression. But having *taken a closer look* at his family history, *it becomes clear* that he has always *looked on the dark side* of things. At present, *he can see* no way out of his depression. *He is looking forward* to *seeing you*, however, and *I regard this* as *a good sign*. It *seems* he was made redundant six weeks ago. He says he finds it difficult *staring at* the same four walls every day. *His view of reality* is becoming somewhat distorted. He is also neglecting his *appearance*, which hardly helps his *self-image* at the moment.

Get the picture? The letter which the CPN team received might have been very different if Ken had, instead, seen Dr V Zyewell's partner, Dr O'Dittrey. Had this been the case, the referral letter might have *sounded* like this:

Letter from Dr O'Dittrey re Mr Ken S Tettik

I was glad to hear, from our telephone conversation the other day, that you are able to offer this man some talking time. It sounds like he has always been rather depressive. Six weeks ago, he was told he was being made redundant. I offered him anti-depressants but he would not hear of it. The mention of counselling, however, seems to have struck a chord with him. It sounds like he is beginning to get rather out of tune with reality. There is also some marital disharmony. I would be glad to hear your opinion, when you have had a chance to sound him out.

The CPN taking on the referral, whichever letter he or she received, would not know the primary representational system of the client in advance. This, however, would become obvious in the initial interview with Ken. Assuming Ken lives up to his name, he would respond best to questions about how he feels, about the sensations and texture of his problems. Trusty therapeutic interventions like, 'How do things look to you right now?' (a favourite of Dr

Zyewell's) would perhaps not elicit as good a response as, 'How do you feel about things right now?' Likewise, one of Dr O'Dittrey's best attempts at empathy, 'It sounds like things have been building up to a crescendo lately', might communicate less empathy to Ken than a statement such as, 'I get the feeling things have been getting harder and harder for you lately'.

After reading these descriptions you will hopefully have a clearer idea of what is meant by kinesthetic, visual and auditory representational systems. Sensitised to these, you may like to consider which of the three is your own primary representational system. Remember that nobody uses only one system but, according to NLP theory, each of us tends to use one or two systems predominantly. Personal interests and occupations are good clues. For example, musicians and linguists may be more likely to have an auditory primary representational system, painters and opticians a visual one.

Those involved in counselling and other interpersonal activities perhaps need to be more aware of their own primary representational system. Such an awareness may be an important element in developing overall self-awareness. It may enable the individual to identify, in turn, the representational systems used by clients and allow for a conscious matching of systems.

As one whose primary representational system seems to be auditory, I earlier used the phrase 'on the same wavelength'. Increased awareness of representational systems promises to improve rapport with clients by demonstrating empathy – you use the same predicates, you speak the same language. If nothing more, it would seem to be a useful aid to empathic communication.

Reflection

Psychiatric nursing students had, at one time, to complete a number of practical assessments. One of these was the 'drug assessment', which usually involved carrying out a medicine round on a ward and being tested on the drugs administered. For example, the assessor would ask what the generic name of a brand-named drug was or vice versa, or what the side-effects of such and such a drug were. It was a good test of a limited body of knowledge, a test of the student's knowledge of 'commonly used drugs in psychiatry'. Knowledge about these drugs was organised into groups of drugs (antidepressants, antipsychotics, anticonvulsants, anxiolytics), and then further broken down into sub-groups (antidepressants consisted of tricyclics and mono-amine oxidase inhibitors; antipsychotics consisted of phenothiazines, butyrophenones and thioxanthenes). Taking this further, examples of thioxanthenes were flupenthixol and zuclopenthixol. A typical 'drugs assessment' might include questions like 'What kind of drug is flupenthixol?', 'What is the other name for amitriptyline?' and 'What are the side-effects of haloperidol?'

Medication seemed a straightforward matter because the 'drug assessment' gave us the false impression that there was a relatively stable body of knowledge that could be grasped, built upon and, ultimately, mastered. In fact, unpredictable things kept happening to this body of knowledge. Suddenly, a drug that you thought you had a good knowledge of would be withdrawn, having been found to be unsafe. Next minute, a new anxiolytic would come onto the market, claiming to be non-addictive. Then a new antidepressant, then a new antipsychotic. The 'drug assessment' was only a moment in time and the fast-moving world of psychopharmacology proved to be in a constant state of flux.

The 1990s saw a puzzling upsurge in depression. Psychologist Oliver James wrote about our 'low Serotonin society' claiming that, despite being richer than we were in the 1950s, our society had become unhappier (James 1998). Other commentators, like psychiatrist David Healy, suspected the pharmaceutical industry of almost 'manufacturing' depression (or at least promoting the diagnosis of it) in order to create a market for their new wave of antidepressants (Healy 1999).

As CPNs, we have had to keep our eye on the ball. In the field of antidepressant treatments alone, we have had to familiarise ourselves with Selective Serotonin Reuptake Inhibitors and, then, dual-action Selective Serotonin Reuptake Inhibitors, Serotonin and Noradrenalin Reuptake Inhibitors, Reversible Inhibitors of Monoamine Oxidase, Noradrenergic and Specific Serotonergic Antidepressants and Noradrenalin Reuptake Inhibitors!

Many of these drugs, when they are first introduced, are referred to as 'atypical' or 'novel' treatments but, as they grow more widely used, they become the mainstream, displacing 'the older treatments'. All that glitters is not gold but a wider range of treatment options, be these pharmacological or psychosocial, is probably a net gain for patients. CPNs, though, need to be able to adapt their practice in order to keep pace with such new developments.

Antidepressant discontinuation syndrome

At the beginning of the 1990s, CPNs began to become aware of patients and their families asking their doctors about Selective Serotonin Reuptake Inhibitors (SSRIs). The SSRI group of antidepressants included four drugs: Fluoxetine, Sertraline, Paroxetine and Fluvoxamine. Some of their popularity seemed to be based on the relative safety of these drugs in the event of an overdose.

The resultant upsurge in SSRI prescribing was a refreshing change to the standard practice of putting the patient on a course of tricyclic antidepressants. Despite the fact that SSRI tablets cost more, it might prove more clinically effective and more cost-effective in the long run to prescribe an SSRI as a first-line treatment, especially since GPs were consistently underprescribing the dosages of the older tricyclics. GPs were quick to see the benefits, both to the patients and to themselves. However, the rise in SSRI prescribing led some to wonder if GPs were not regarding them as a new panacea, just as benzodiazepines had once been seen as a cure-all for every form of anxiety and depression.

CPNs began to observe symptoms when patients stopped SSRIs. We had noticed patients complaining of increased anxiety, insomnia, headaches, nausea. Were they suffering a relapse or a withdrawal? Had CPNs found the Achilles' heel of SSRIs? Had these patients developed a dependency on their antidepressants that meant they relapsed upon stopping treatment? We had been telling our patients that they were wrong to confuse antidepressants with benzodiazepines. We had repeatedly stated that antidepressants were not addictive. Had we been misleading our patients?

In October 1998, the European College of Neuropsychopharmacology met in Paris and heard preliminary results from a new survey into GPs' knowledge of Antidepressant Discontinuation Syndrome. There, Dr Peter Haddad commented:

> There is overwhelming evidence that antidepressants are not drugs of dependence. Antidepressants are the same as many drugs used extensively in modern medicine, such as beta-blockers or diuretics. If a patient's long term treatment is abruptly stopped, there is always a readjustment period that can lead to transient symptoms.

It comes, then, as a great reassurance to learn that discontinuation syndrome is not simply a euphemism for withdrawal symptoms. However, awareness of discontinuation syndrome has implications for mental health professionals. Dr Haddad's remarks remind us that these symptoms are transient but the difficulty for CPNs, doctors and their patients lies in determining when the symptoms are part of discontinuation syndrome and when they are early warning signs of relapse.

Patients may need as much monitoring at the end of their treatment as at the beginning. This may require a considerable shift in working practice in that, up till now, we have tended to taper off our intervention just as medication is reduced because the patient's condition has improved. The idea is to reduce dependency on psychiatric services gradually as the illness improves.

If we are to anticipate the possibility of discontinuation symptoms, perhaps we should plan to be more available for patients as they gradually reduce their medication. In this way, we can support patients through a potentially difficult period and, at the same time, check that they have not stopped treatment too early. Antidepressant treatment should not be reinstated unnecessarily if the patient is experiencing discontinuation syndrome but, if they are re-presenting with a depressive illness, early intervention would be helpful.

Alternatively, in the interests of reducing dependency on CPN services, perhaps it should be the prescriber – be it the GP or psychiatrist – who closely monitors the end of treatment, allowing the CPN to disengage naturally. In the knowledge that antidepressants are not drugs of dependence, our aim must remain to promote the psychological and social independence of our patients.

Reflection

In parallel with the new wave of antidepressants, the pharmaceutical industry has been busy over the last decade introducing 'atypical' antipsychotics. Clozapine, risperidone, sertindole (now suspended), olanzapine, amisulpride, quetiapine and zotepine have appeared. Some of these drugs are entirely new, others relative newcomers to the UK. What is interesting, from the point of view of community psychiatric nursing, is, not just their mode of action, but their mode of delivery. The fact that all of these drugs are oral preparations and none of them, so far, is available in the form of a depot injection has an impact on the role of the CPN. Of course, I am not suggesting that CPNs are lost without the ability to give injections. It has been noted elsewhere, though, that Sladden (1979) referred to the administration of depot injections as the main raison d'être of CPNs (see Chapter 3). However, if medication is the mainstay of treatment for illnesses such as schizophrenia, and if this medication is to be in tablet rather than injection form, it changes the relationship between CPN and patient. It involves a greater sharing of power between the two and gives the patient greater responsibility to manage their own illness. This can be both risky and tremendously liberating (see Chapter 5).

In the past year I have seen a number of my patients 'switched' from traditional depot injections to 'atypicals'. In fact, in some cases, the oral medication has been a 'typical' oral medication, such as sulpiride, which seems to have enjoyed a resurgence thanks to the trend away from injections. Some of these patients have quickly relapsed because, given the freedom and responsibility to take their own medicine, they have 'chosen' to stop treatment. The word 'chosen' is used advisedly because, where motivation and insight into the illness is variable, it is debatable how much this is a conscious choice.

Some CPNs have recognised that the control of the depot injection cannot be removed without setting up additional means of support, to bolster motivation and insight, so that patients and their carers can work in partnership. Psychosocial interventions take on a central importance. Education, family interventions and carers' groups, for example, are needed to complement the use of medication.

CPNs will probably always be needed to administer depot injections for a certain group of patients. Many patients, however, will be able to remain well on oral medication so long as they are given education about their illness and its management. CPNs are well placed, perhaps even best placed, to ensure that patients and families receive this. As a profession, we should be careful not to take on the lion's share of this great task but our fair share. Clarke worries that, for psychiatric nurses working with serious and enduring illness:

> interventions are either going to be cognitive-behaviourist in nature, thus edging nursing towards a psychological mode of practice, or they are going

to be of a nature which will return nurses to the role of interminable second-fiddle to a medical speciality which enduringly controls diagnosis and prescription.

(Clarke 1999: 5)

This may amount to saying that the CPN is either a 'poor man's psychologist' or a doctor's handmaiden. I think we should be neither but there is a major role for the CPN that involves having an excellent knowledge of medication relevant to mental health, and excellent knowledge and skills in psychosocial interventions. This combination is rare among other disciplines. It may be rare among CPNs at present. Focusing overmuch on either medication or psychosocial interventions will create an imbalanced practitioner who is, perhaps, 'neither one thing nor the other'. There is no need for a 'poor man's psychologist' or a doctor's handmaiden. A good psychologist and a good psychiatrist will do fine, and a good CPN, working in partnership with the other disciplines, will do better still.

Psychosocial interventions should not remain 'atypical'. They need to be seen as a core part of the service CPNs provide. Medication cannot be brushed under the carpet and CPNs need to keep updated because today's 'atypical' treatments become tomorrow's 'typical' treatments. There is a greater choice of interventions, which can be of great benefit to patients. It is the CPN's responsibility to share this choice in a creative and thoughtful way.

Schizophrenia and atypical antipsychotics

In this age of community care, families are expected to look after people with mental illness. Some professional help is available, of course. Medication is prescribed, psychiatrists are seen in out-patients' clinics, a CPN may visit. Still, families are largely expected to care for people with schizophrenia without training, without pay, without a break. What causes schizophrenia – a question many patients and their families want answered – remains open to debate. For want of a clear understanding of the causes, the management of schizophrenia has tended to focus on treatment of the symptoms, prevention of relapse and minimising the long-term consequences of the illness.

Two forms of intervention have been shown to be helpful in schizophrenia. These are medication and family therapy. While the use of medication is widespread, family work and other psychosocial interventions are generally less available. Non-compliance with treatment tends to lead to relapse and more frequent hospitalisation. The disruption this causes to the lives of patients and their families should not be underestimated.

Family interventions (see Chapter 10) have been shown to prevent relapse, reduce hospitalisations and improve compliance with medication (Mari *et al.* 1997). Family interventions do not and cannot work in isolation, however. They rely on the patient being well enough to take part. For this reason, medication remains a mainstay of treatment.

Gournay and Gray (1998) argued that the introduction of novel antipsychotics heralded a revolution in the drug treatment of schizophrenia. The drugs to which they were referring were clozapine, risperidone, sertindole and olanzapine. Sertindole has since been suspended but the list of new atypical antipsychotics continues to grow with amisulpride, quetiapine and zotepine being added to the formulary. Gournay and Gray cited evidence that atypicals 'may have superior outcome measures over the traditional compounds, may help patients who previously failed to respond to the traditional drugs, but may also be more acceptable to patients' (Gournay and Gray 1998: 21–22). This is certainly borne out, for example, by a key paper on the long-term safety and efficacy of amisulpride (Colonna *et al.* 2000).

For many patients the depot injection is a very aversive experience. However skilled the nurse, receiving an injection remains a potentially painful experience for many. It can be embarrassing (given the preferred site of injection) and can be perceived as controlling, disempowering, even punitive. For some, then, it is no wonder continued maintenance depot treatment appears an unattractive option. Even in the most insightful of patients, this can lead to noncompliance. The option of oral medication for certain patients is liberating and is likely to promote compliance in those individuals who are averse to the traditional depot injection.

Of course, it could be said that the option of oral medication has always existed. However, the advantage of atypicals is that they tend to produce therapeutic effects with less risk of producing extrapyramidal side-effects. It is often these side-effects (or sometimes worries of developing these side-effects or memories of previous bad experiences) that discourage patients from accepting antipsychotic medication in any form. It is important to point out that atypicals are not without their side-effects (e.g. weight gain to a greater or lesser extent, that may have long-term implications for health).

One further aspect of treatment that may reduce compliance is the need for what might be seen as more invasive forms of monitoring, such as blood tests. The need for regular blood tests could be perceived by patients as hardly preferable to injections. Though perhaps less embarrassing, they may be painful and may also be viewed as an inconvenience if they require attendance at clinics.

It must be recognised that compliance with oral therapy may be poor in patients with persecutory delusional beliefs extending to the medication, and those with poor insight or limited motivation. However, any medication that can be *taken* orally, rather than *given* intramuscularly, has the distinctive feature of restoring control of the illness to the patient. This implies a trusting collaborative relationship between patient and professionals and, preferably, between patient, professionals and the patient's family.

It must be acknowledged that sometimes this is not possible; occasionally, healthcare workers have to act in a more paternalistic or authoritative way. However, for many patients a working partnership with the CPN, doctor and family is perfectly possible. Medication that avoids the need for injections or blood tests and that minimises the risk of side-effects is likely to be more acceptable.

A final word needs to be said about negative symptoms. Professionals are sometimes surprised to find that it is these, and not the positive symptoms, with which families have the greatest difficulty coping. Positive symptoms are a clear reminder of the illness and are often assertively treated by health professionals. It is the lack of motivation, the staying in bed for hours, the difficulty holding conversation, which lead to frustration and despair.

There is some evidence that certain atypicals may also improve the negative, as well as the positive, symptoms of schizophrenia (Dratcu 2000). This is an encouraging sign for patients and their families. If both positive and negative symptoms can be improved with medication, working alongside psychosocial interventions, the outlook for people with schizophrenia can only be brighter.

8   Reintegration through creativity

Reflection

Re-reading 'Creative arts as therapy' more than a decade after it was first published, I am struck by just how much has changed. The article compares two
different types of musical activity. One type was based on my experiences as a
student nurse at Shelton Hospital in Shrewsbury. Shelton Hospital opened in
1845, as the New Shropshire Lunatic Asylum. I trained there from 1983 to
1986 and now realise I caught the very last glimpses of the end of an era.

It was part of my job, as a student nurse, to escort patients to various
activities around the hospital. There was an industrial therapy department
(where I packed hair-curlers and wired lamp-fittings with patients who were
much more skilled than I at these tasks). There was a recreational therapy
department, where I improved my game of pool, while discussing heavy-
metal music, and experimented with some very early versions of electronic
games. There was a newly built occupational therapy department that
employed a professional art therapist. Still, many of the long-stay patients
were led to the main hall where various social activities (like the singalong
session described) took place.

The second type of musical activity described is based on my experience at
West Bank Day Hospital in Telford. Here was a place that seemed to revel in
group work of all sorts. Its philosophy was rather like a therapeutic community and it used drama, art and all kinds of group work in a very enlightened
way. As a student, I was given quite a free rein here to try out my idea of a
'music workshop' group.

The difference in atmosphere between the grandeur and tradition of the
hospital and the seeming radicalism of the day hospital is almost a metaphor
for the shift from long-stay in-patient care to community care. Nurses who
remember the old hospitals, although perhaps not wishing to return to cus-
todial care, are at times nostalgic about what may have been lost in the
modernisation. Books of old photographs are now published. Morris has written an excellent history of Shelton Hospital (Morris 1998), while Jocelyn
Goddard's *Mixed Feelings* pays similar tribute to Oxfordshire's Littlemore
Hospital (Goddard 1996).

Gone are many of the recreational and industrial therapy departments along with the long-stay wards. Gone also, though, are many of the beautiful gardens and cricket pavilions around which nurses like me would stroll and chat with patients. In-patients in modern psychiatric hospitals often have nowhere pleasant to roam on the hospital site – only overcrowded car parks or little concrete-slabbed patios.

What in-patients do have more of nowadays are visitors, who seemed rather scarce on the long-stay wards. Some families had disowned their 'lunatic' relatives. Some were forgotten. Some had been orphans, others prisoners of war, shifted halfway across Europe, barely able to speak English. Some had relatives living in town but mental hospitals were built deliberately far from town.

It is worth recalling our mixed feelings about the history and tradition of psychiatric nursing. It is also worth considering how the art and science of nursing can promote creativity as a means to mental health. My impression is that the capacity of the arts to help reintegrate individuals into groups, communities and society is still not appreciated fully.

Creative arts as therapy

In a society geared towards industrialisation and economic growth, and informed by hard science, it is easy to view creative art as an indulgence. Artists are thus marginalised and are seen, like homeless or mentally ill people, as outside the mainstream of society – perhaps as an encumbrance. While considering this, it might be worth asking why governments who seem to underinvest in health, education, housing and welfare also appear to underinvest in the arts.

If scientific evidence is used to substantiate advertisers' claims on everything from washing powder to superglue, it is no wonder qualities like creativity and spontaneity are undervalued. Nursing might have been in the vanguard of exploring the exciting potential of artistic therapies. With its traditional close allegiance to medicine, however, nursing has tended to think scientifically and mechanistically, rather than artistically or imaginatively. Society expects nurses to be solid, reliable, practical and predictable.

In an ethos where science is the new religion, the hallmark of serious intellect and respectability, it is understandable that nursing, in struggling to assert itself as a *real* profession, emphasises scientifically measurable aspects of its work. No matter how holistic, humanistic or patient-centred nurses try to be, the profession cannot overcome its overemphasis on science. Even the nursing process is part of this self-mystification, reducing a person's suffering to so many enumerated problems which can be processed. The prominence given to research is another example of this. Every aspect of caring must be analysed and the findings collated. How can the arts flourish as a therapeutic tool in such an atmosphere? Yet, there are many ways in which creative arts can be used in practical therapeutic settings. Consider the following two scenes:

- **Scene one** – a traditional psychiatric hospital. A large group of long-stay patients is gathered, sitting in rows in the main hall. They are there to join in a singalong session led by a lady playing the piano. A box of percussion instruments is passed round and patients are encouraged to take out tambourines and maracas to accompany *The Skye Boat Song* and *Daisy, Daisy.*
- **Scene two** – a modern psychiatric day hospital. In a small but spacious room, six patients and two nurses are grouped in a rough circle. An anxious, agoraphobic lady is singing *The Hills are Alive with the Sound of Music.* It is her turn to sing. In another exercise, a middle-aged man, treated like an overgrown child by his parents, expresses his unspeakable anger and frustration with an isolated, resonating beat on a tambourine.

In scene one the 'music therapy' on offer in the main hall is seen primarily as a recreational activity. It is also communal, in the same way that bingo and even church services were regarded in older psychiatric hospitals. They are a way of getting patients together. To this extent, the therapeutic aspects of this activity are that the patient has a change of scene, some time away from the ward, and may be sufficiently inspired to join in and have fun. Unfortunately, many patients attend under duress. Unmotivated and withdrawn, as many long-stay patients are, an entertainment of this kind is the last place they would choose to go were they not cajoled by the nurses. Often, the choice of music and its style of presentation would remind many of schooldays, and being asked to play a triangle will only reinforce this perception.

Essentially, such use of an art form is passive. Despite being asked to participate, the patients are on the receiving end of a prescribed treatment. If they sing or play along at all, it is merely audience participation.

Of course, there is nothing intrinsically wrong with being passive in our artistic involvement. Nearly everybody is. Most people read books rather than write them. There are far more people listening to radios than there are songwriters. Just as in everyday life the passive enjoyment of the arts is wonderful, in health care settings this way of being involved is also undoubtedly therapeutic.

Hospital radio is a widespread and hugely appreciated form of passive music therapy. Patients' libraries are a welcome literary lifeline for many. Some hospitals even experiment with exhibitions of paintings to enliven their clinically cold corridors. All this must make time spent in hospital more enjoyable for everyone. It must, by the same token, be helping patients get better but what if this is just the tip of the iceberg? What if nurses could not only escort patients to enjoy artistic activities but could actually organise those activities themselves? And what if, with our ideals of helping patients to help themselves, nurses could facilitate the creative use of the arts by the patients themselves?

In scene two, just by a change of location, the spectre of institutionalisation is immediately shaken off. In a smaller community setting, patients (or clients) would probably receive a more individualised kind of care to meet their own personal needs, rather than primarily those of society. The room is not the impersonal hall but a more intimate place, conducive to social interaction as opposed to the isolation of a crowd. The group of patients is of a manageable size, made up of people with a special interest in exploring their feelings through an art form. They do not necessarily have any special skills in the techniques of that form. Again, the nurses working with them will have an enthusiasm for music, art, writing, drama or whatever it may be. They are not merely attendants at the event, or escorts, but are integral members of the group, which has an identity promoted and symbolised by its grouping into a circle rather than rows. The patients are not merely the audience but are performers, audience, perhaps even critics of the session.

The scope of the group depends on the motivation and imagination of its members. However, a music therapy session like the one described in scene two could be used as a vehicle for desensitisation, relaxation, social skills training, assertiveness and self-awareness.

What is really happening in scene two is a kind of group therapy. One might say it is group therapy set to music. The effect could be the same whether it was dance, drama, art or creative writing. In addition to the therapeutic effects of the art form itself, the participants would be gaining the therapeutic benefits of working in a group.

Nurses in various settings may find themselves working, not with individuals in isolation, but with groups of patients. I would like to suggest that, for nurses considering how they might best use a creative art with their patients, the effects can be enhanced by organising it as a group activity. Yalom (1986) identified eleven 'curative factors' that come into play, to a greater or lesser extent, in any therapeutic group situation. These include such factors as the instillation of hope, interpersonal learning and group cohesiveness.

Certainly, working in groups has benefits. A creative art can be used as a vehicle for a kind of incidental group therapy, which patients may find less threatening than the more conventional form of talking and listening as a group. This is particularly true of patients who have difficulty expressing themselves verbally, whether due to physiological or psychological causes.

Some creative arts therapies have evolved into professions in their own right, with their own professional associations, recognised training courses and qualifications. Taken together, they form a broad spectrum covering all the various art forms, in all their various styles. On the one hand, there are academically qualified or classically trained artists who have gone on to train in using their art as therapy. On the other, there are formally trained artists who take posts as artists-in-residence in various health care settings.

In addition to these two groups, there are health professionals who use a creative art in their work and may go on to take some formal training in their chosen art as therapy. For instance, while there are some professional drama therapists, nurses and other professionals are increasingly using drama therapy as an additional tool in their work. Organisations, such as the British Association of Drama Therapy, Sesame and the British Psychodrama Association, provide various types of training to help nurses integrate the use of drama in this way. Likewise, the British Society for Music Therapy runs short courses for nurses wishing to integrate music therapy into their work. The society disseminates information and organises conferences, workshops and meetings. Membership is open to all who have an interest in music therapy in the UK and worldwide.

Perhaps the least popular of performing arts therapies in the UK is dance therapy. It has, nevertheless, continued to gain status in the United States since its emergence there in the 1940s. Dance therapy is based on the concept of body–mind integration and the belief that awareness of the body leads to awareness of feelings.

Creative writing may seem a very private, unsociable activity but it can also be good therapy. As well as being an ideal means of self-help through self-expression, by reading aloud, and giving and receiving group feedback, creative writing can effectively be used as a form of group therapy.

Reflection

The article 'Creative arts as therapy' acknowledges the reality that, where the arts are used in a therapeutic way in mental health, it is often psychiatric nurses (or social workers or occupational therapists) rather than professional arts therapists who are facilitating this. The article sets out to encourage this trend, which I believe is good for patients and for nurses. My intention was not to upset or alienate professional arts therapists. In fact, I hope that the growth in arts activities led by nurses and others promotes a greater recognition of the need for arts therapists and, come to that, the need for professional artists. However, this can be an area of tension between professions so I felt I had to be diplomatic in how I described my music workshops.

The article 'Sounds good' describes the process of setting up music workshops and explores the underlying issues relating to music, therapy and music therapy, with due deference to professional music therapists. Unfortunately, I still managed to upset at least one music therapist who wrote a letter to *Nursing Times* criticising my comments about the lack of a coherent evidence-base for music therapy. I was trying to say that, as regards a theory underpinning our work in mental health, nursing and music therapy are in the same, rather shaky, boat. Of course, having a questionable theoretical base does not diminish a profession, though many nurses have acted as if their life depended on developing a theory or a body of knowledge. Perhaps this is driven by an unfounded belief that the 'proper professions' (and, of course, medicine is the one nursing loves to hate most) have an unquestionable scientific foundation. The point is that all theory/knowledge/science/evidence is open to question. There is room for different kinds of evidence and, despite the fashion for evidence-based practice (which is no bad thing), surely creative arts therapies, just like psychiatric nursing, are more 'healing arts' than they are 'scientific treatments'.

Health professionals tend to worry about these questions a great deal but patients (the users of the service) may care less about the theory and more about the outcome. Thus, one member of the Music Workshop Project told me the project's activities are not really comparable with music therapy. He had experienced both; having been a patient in a music therapy group run by a professional music therapist and a participant in our music workshop. He reminded me that patients are not *referred* to the project for *music therapy*. They may be invited by a mental health worker or another member of the group, or may simply choose to come along and take part in a workshop. The workshops often function more like a self-help group, or just a recreational group activity, or simply 'a bit of fun'. The fact that participants seem to find them 'therapeutic' in some sense is a happy accident – serendipity rather than treatment.

Sounds good – establishing therapeutic music groups in community mental health settings

Music at the Oasis

An oasis is an area of calm in the midst of turbulence. We identified a need for such a place in our community for young people with mental health problems. So, the Oasis Group was born, intended as a meeting place for people aged from 18 to 30 who have mental health problems, offering activities appropriate to their age group.

The group – the result of an imaginative multi-agency collaboration – originally involved mental health charity MIND, the local social services department and the youth service. It is supported by CPNs and mental health social workers. Part of the original aim of the Oasis Group was to provide sports and arts activities that would be of particular interest to young people with mental health problems. One of the activities on offer is the monthly music workshop.

In the early days of the Oasis, the one-hour lunchtime music workshops were led by myself and a social worker from a local rehabilitation hostel. A range of musical instruments (mainly percussion) was provided and all members were encouraged to try improvisation. The workshops, developed from a series of closed groups, are described below. To fully understand how the format of these sessions was arrived at, however, it is first necessary to explore some of the concepts underpinning music therapy.

Definitions of music therapy

A pioneer of music therapy, Alvin, defined it as 'the controlled use of music in the treatment, rehabilitation, education and training of children and adults suffering from physical, mental or emotional disorder' (Alvin 1975: 4). Another definition, a synthesis of several others, is provided by Bunt who says that music therapy is 'the use of organised sounds and music within an evolving relationship between client and therapist to support and encourage physical, mental, social and emotional well-being' (Bunt 1994: 8).

Musicians, music therapists and therapists

Some of the definitions of music therapy suggest that it is a skill to be practised by trained practitioners. Words such as specialised and systematic might seem to imply that only a trained, qualified or professional music therapist is able to practise true music therapy. However, most definitions are less exclusive and would embrace looser concepts, such as 'therapeutic music-making' and 'music *in* therapy', alongside 'music *as* therapy' (Benenzon 1981). While those concerned with the development of music therapy into a profession will demand a high standard of musicianship or academic qualification in music as a prerequisite to training as a therapist, others see the therapist element as more important than the musician element. Benenzon, for example, believes that a music therapist need not be a trained musician (ibid.).

Music therapy, nursing and research

Like nursing, music therapy was, from its inception, not a particularly research-based profession. Nursing has, in the past, been criticised for lacking a sound theoretical base and for borrowing theoretical concepts and models from medicine. It could, similarly, be argued that – although musical theory is well established – music therapy has lacked a distinct body of research and, like other creative arts therapies, has tended to draw heavily on theories from psychology and psychotherapy. In recent years, music therapists have made efforts to generate a body of research unique to itself (Bunt 1994) and, in this way, there is a parallel process going on in both the nursing and music therapy professions.

What business do mental health nurses have with music therapy?

It could be argued that such activities are peripheral to nursing and should have a low priority. However, if it is accepted that music has a role in the treatment, rehabilitation and education of adults with mental or emotional disorder (Alvin 1975), or in supporting and encouraging mental, social and emotional well-being (Bunt 1994), then it follows that this is very much an area in which mental health nurses ought to be involved.

Furthermore, if therapeutic skill is recognised as equal, if not greater, in importance than musical accomplishment, there is no impediment to mental health nurses being involved in music therapy. If it offends professional music therapists to think that those with less specialised training, or less musical expertise, might claim to practise music therapy, phrases like 'the therapeutic use of music' or 'therapeutic music-making' can be used. Nurses need not, nor should they, claim to *be* music therapists. What is important in the case of community psychiatric nurses is that, whatever their therapeutic musical activities are called, they should take place *in the community*.

What is a music workshop?

Having run similar groups in day hospitals before becoming a CPN, I find referring to the group as a 'music workshop' helpful because clients often find the concept of a workshop acceptable, where an invitation to take part in a music therapy group might be challenging. Above all, the term evokes a sense of experimentation, of work in progress, that will perhaps never be completed. It implies work, rather than pure recreation, and that music will be made rather than passively received. It is also intended to convey a sense that the 'therapists' are not necessarily 'experts' and that they too are interested in the experiment. Table 8.1 outlines a blueprint for music workshops.

Table 8.1 Blueprint for music workshops

Size of group:
One–two therapist(s) and four–six patients/clients
Duration and frequency of meeting:
One hour, once a week, for eight weeks
Aims of group:
• To encourage interpersonal communication
• To learn to explore and express feelings and moods through music
• To promote spontaneity, creativity and 'playfulness' as a means of relaxation and recreation

---

Criteria for admission to the group

Clients need not have any ability in playing any particular instrument nor any knowledge of musical theory. Clients should be willing to experiment with making music (or sounds) on a range of instruments, in a group setting. Those who do have some ability in playing an instrument might like to consider the group as an opportunity to learn new ways of exploring music with non-musicians.

What the group is and is not about

Music workshops are not designed for competent musicians. They do not aim to teach people to be competent musicians but rather aim to promote an interest in making music and exploring its potential for personal expression and interpersonal communication. The groups are not for listening passively to music but for actively creating it.

At times, group members will be given the opportunity to discuss their music and their feelings about the music, themselves and each other. The focus of the group is twofold – for clients to experience the therapeutic effects of being creative and to develop interpersonal skills through group-work.

Evaluation

The closed group ran for eight weeks in 1995 and was based at the Community House, a building attached to a local social services hostel for the rehabilitation of people with mental health problems. We attempted to target people with more severe mental illness but a mixture of severely and less-severely ill people eventually attended.

We also wanted to achieve a gender balance but most members were men. During the course of the eight weeks, members began dropping out and at the end of the sessions only two young men remained. Interestingly, one was relatively well and was a fairly accomplished musician, while the other was a young man with a diagnosis of schizophrenia whose ambition was to 'learn a few chords' on his guitar. Nevertheless, the cohesion between these two was remarkably good. In order to have some objective evaluation of the work-shops, we adapted a questionnaire normally used to evaluate anxiety-management groups. Table 8.2 shows some of the comments received.

Table 8.2 Workshop members' comments

'I expected the group to be a bit of a free-for-all music session.'
'I thought I might be taught a few chords, which did happen in the last session.'
'It was as if I was releasing some emotions, which was good when we were all joining in.'
'I found the feeling of belonging to something helpful.'
'I definitely feel slightly more outgoing.'
'It was good to have a laugh occasionally, which we did when we got to know each other.'
'More than anything it was enjoyable.'
'It was very interesting, playing music together. I have never done this before.'

Moving the closed group out into 'the community'

Towards the end of the eight weeks, group members expressed a desire to con-tinue the music workshops in some form. We agreed that a monthly session should be set up to take place at the Oasis Group. Oasis seemed an ideal place for members of the closed group to share their music therapy experience with a wider group. The term 'audience' has been consciously avoided here, since it is important that clients feel they are participating mutually rather than performing or 'in the spotlight'.

Integrating members of the closed music workshop group into a monthly open music workshop session at the Oasis Group has widened the participants' social horizons. Closed groups can be seen as a sort of 'training ground' for clients who wish to take a leading role in the Oasis music workshop sessions.

The furtherance of music workshops

Our plan was to continue taking referrals from CPNs, social workers and outreach workers, so that the focus remained on patients and clients living in the community. Community workers were also encouraged to invite their clients to try out the open sessions at the Oasis Group. In addition, I became involved in teaching other nurses how to use music therapeutically in groups.

The teaching and the therapeutic work itself was based on firmly held and, perhaps, unfashionable beliefs. These included the assumption that mental health nursing needs to be creative and innovative in order to meet the needs of people (and, particularly, *young* people) with mental health problems. There often seems to be a lack of resources targeted at young people with mental illness.

All the creative arts, and music especially, are particularly relevant to this client group and, so, should not be regarded as a peripheral luxury. Because music is a powerful therapeutic tool, activities involving music and music therapy could play a much more important role in the future planning of mental health services.

Reflection

I have noticed, in re-reading the articles 'Sounds good' and 'Song sung blue', a tone which implies the Project is a piece of work successfully brought to completion, its potential fully realised. I had carried with me the idea of the experimental music group that I had first tried out as a student nurse at the day hospital in Telford. As a staff nurse at Kidderminster Day Hospital I had reinvented the music workshops and, for a while after I had left, they employed a professional music therapist. I think this proves my point that nurse-led arts activities promote the creative arts therapy professions, rather than competing with them.

'Sounds good' describes how the Oasis drop-in, and the music workshop element of it, were created to meet a specific service need. Managers of mental health services will view such initiatives as innovative if they successfully meet such a need, or plain eccentric if they do not! However, setting up new schemes must, in some way, satisfy our own needs and not just those of our patients if we are to find the motivation to bring them to fruition. This is not to say that we are putting our own needs before the patients' but that successful projects meet the needs of everyone involved.

When I became a CPN, I suppose I missed (and looked for) opportunities to continue group work in community settings (see Chapter 2). The music workshops at the Community House had developed into a more autonomous group at the Oasis. I had envisaged running one or two more closed groups to 'feed into' the open group. (This is the 'training ground' idea mentioned in 'Sounds good'.) I think I had an idea that, at some point, the music workshop sessions at the Oasis might become a sort of self-help group. I did not imagine that the workshops would mature into a self-sustaining *project* like the Music Workshop Project, described in 'Song sung blue'.

The peculiar thing about the Project is that it never seems to stop evolving. At the time of writing 'Song sung blue', we were releasing a CD compilation album, *Organised Chaos*, and launching our own website (www.musicworkshop.org.uk). I keep thinking we must have reached a plateau but, driven very much by the wishes of the group members, the Project goes on developing in new directions, a constant source of professional challenge and stimulation.

My assumption that the Project had more or less realised its full potential was, therefore, misplaced. After recording a few tracks, people naturally think about collecting them together as a compilation album. After doing this, they naturally want to release that album. To release an album, you have to design the sleeve. I am ashamed to admit that I underestimated the talent and energy of this group of people to produce a finished product – an album and a website, and then to want to go on to produce a further album, all the time continuing to attend monthly workshops in which the most remarkable music is generated.

The members of the Music Workshop Project are a privilege to work with and have achieved so much for which they should be proud. Instead, faced with the stigma that blights people with mental health problems, they are wary of the publicity their work invites. I have found myself in the role of spokesperson for the group when dealing with the media attention we have attracted. Once or twice, professional photographers have arrived to photograph group members for a newspaper or a magazine. I have carefully asked participants to give written consent for their photograph to be published and for them to be identified with the Project in this way. Often, it seems people are proud of the Project but embarrassed that they will be publicly identified as someone with a mental health problem. A major task ahead for all of us is to find ways of working with the users of mental health services to break down the stigma of mental illness. How do we celebrate the achievements of people with mental health problems without causing embarrassment? Do we ignore the 'mental health label' altogether or would this only be doing a greater disservice to the mentally ill?

Song sung blue – how the Music Workshop Project has developed

From closed group to open session

At times, the original music workshop group had allowed group members the opportunity to discuss their music, and their feelings about the music, themselves and each other. As the workshop sessions have become more 'open', with people dropping in and out, this has necessarily changed. Recently, the group's fluid membership has meant there is perhaps less trust and so less of a willingness to disclose feelings. Nowadays, workshops are less exploratory and are more involved with the business of simply making music.

Increasing user-involvement

The Project was the subject of a workshop I presented at the 1996 Community Psychiatric Nurses' Association (CPNA) conference in Hull. On the strength of this, I was invited to write the article for *Nursing Times*, which became 'Sounds good'. Photographs of project members appeared alongside the article and on the front cover of the magazine on World Mental Health Day 1996. One project member was so encouraged by the media attention he agreed to take on the role of fellow co-ordinator and became actively involved in promoting the Project by writing articles for magazines, and by applying for funding to expand the group's musical activity.

Music workshops for the Millennium

After the excitement of a little media attention, we decided to apply for funding from various bodies in order to purchase some more musical instruments and equipment. Those members of the group who were competent musicians felt they would like the opportunity to record their music to a high standard. We were delighted to receive an award from the Mind Millennium Fund, which has already enabled us to purchase a very sophisticated keyboard and a multi-track mini-disc portable recording machine. Some group members are now making recordings of their own compositions. The award has also allowed us, for the first time, to have high-quality recordings of the improvisations that take place in the music workshop sessions.

An environmentally friendly project

As well as purchasing new equipment with the Mind Millennium Fund grant, the Project was successful in making a bid for a 'GreenGrant'. These grants were made in 1998 by Wyre Forest District Council for environmentally friendly projects in the Wyre Forest area. The council was particularly impressed by the Project's involvement with 'an under-represented group within our community' (i.e. people with mental health problems) and by the 'sustainability' of our proposal to recycle and restore unwanted musical instruments donated by the public for re-use by the Project. This involves the whole community in an environmental task that promotes positive mental health. As well as reducing stigma by bringing the public into contact with mental health services, it also provides skills training in instrument restoration for people with mental health problems.

The local press were quick to publicise our recycling efforts and success with the Mind Millennium Fund. Project members drafted letters to the local paper, photographers were dispatched to photograph a workshop full of broken guitars and keyboards. BBC Radio Hereford and Worcester discussed our work in a live 'phone-in'.

Members of the public kindly brought their unwanted instruments to D Block – the mental health department of Kidderminster General Hospital. Those instruments that needed repairing were worked on by people with mental health problems at two workshops – one at the hospital, the other at the social services day centre. Once restored, they are played by members of the Project, at the Oasis drop-in.

International recognition

In 1998 the project achieved international recognition as the only UK winner of the Lilly Schizophrenia Reintegration Award. As co-ordinator of the project I was invited to attend the award ceremony in Geneva, part of the World Psychiatric Association's (WPA's) European conference. We received a certificate of excellence and a commemorative trophy along with a grant for US$5,000 (about £3,000) to help further develop the work of the Project.

This prestigious award programme was set up in 1995 by Eli Lilly and Company, with the aim of recognising outstanding achievement and innovation in helping people with schizophrenia and related disorders to overcome the barriers to reintegrating back into society (see Chapter 9). Winners were selected by an independent judging panel of leading European experts, including Professor Heinz Katschnig, a psychiatrist from Vienna, and Dr Thomas Stuttaford, a prominent medical journalist who writes for *The Times*. Their selection of the winners was based on both the innovative approach and the success of the projects.

Local, national and international recognition has been accompanied by plenty of media interest in the Project. Newspapers and magazines have carried photographs and articles, and I was interviewed on BBC Radio Hereford and Worcester on World Mental Health Day. All this has helped to present a positive image of mental illness in the media and has boosted the confidence of group members.

Service users have become actively involved in the organisation and planning of the group, they have continued to publish articles and to design promotional materials. Group members were busy throughout 1999 recording their music and went on to produce and release the compilation album *Organised Chaos* in 2000.

Conclusion

Project members did not expect to see their photographs on the cover of national magazines, nor to hear their work discussed on local radio. For those non-musician members, the Project is simply a good night out or just a good way of 'letting off steam'. Some of them aspire to take their music more seriously and are learning or improving their skills on instruments donated to the Project. For those members of the Project who are proficient musicians, it is a dream come true – they have the chance to make professional-quality recordings, to do multi-tracking and to arrange their compositions, and to promote their music beyond the bounds of the Music Workshop Project.

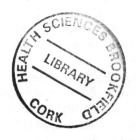

9   True colours
Working with primary care

Reflection

In Chapter 2, I described a little disagreement I once had with a practice manager about the accuracy of information our CPN department were supplying. I was irritated by the obsession with receiving quantitative information and the apparent disregard for the quality of the work. This was against a background of increasing market forces in the NHS. Trust status for health authorities, followed by fundholding status for GP surgeries, seemed to bring out the worst in some health care workers. One GP, in the forefront of fundholding autonomy, angrily expressed his belief that the policy of encouraging patients on lithium to attend our local day hospital's lithium clinic was an example of the consultant psychiatrists' empire-building. In this competitive atmosphere, primary and secondary care workers often become polarised, blaming each other for being too inflexible, or not productive enough, or not communicative enough, or not accurate in their giving of information.

Like the legendary battles between night shift and day shift on some hospital wards, a battle is often enacted between primary and secondary care, where shortcomings or things beyond our control are projected on to the other camp. Resistance to change is normal but the culture of GP fundholding meant that some CPNs were dragged (almost kicking and screaming) into a closer relationship with primary care. The early days of my own experience of this form the subject for 'Too close for comfort?'. Now, it reads as an essay in the management of change and readers may detect signs of separation anxiety in this rather bitter little article. I think I was as angry at being 'abandoned' by secondary care as I was apprehensive about being assimilated – like a victim of the Borg in *Star Trek* – into primary care.

Of course, things have improved since the 'teething problems' described here. This is not so much because I have conformed to primary care's ways. Nor is it that the primary care staff have become tremendously insightful into my working practices or the nature of mental illness and its treatment. We have, no doubt, educated one another to some extent. I have recognised that mental health is not a great priority to many primary care staff (in fact, they often have an attitude closer to that of the general public than that of mental health professionals). They have recognised that I am not 'their' CPN in the old-fashioned way that some GPs seem to have ownership of nursing staff directly employed by practices. We have come to an accommodation but I think this has more to do with the changing social and political backdrop.

More recent government policy has given CPNs 'permission' to focus on severe and enduring mental illness and to concern themselves with evidence-based interventions, such as working with families to improve outcomes in psychosis (see Chapter 10). Meanwhile, GPs and other primary care staff are becoming more confident and more willing to treat psychological illness without always involving the CPN. As much as government policy, perhaps the introduction of newer antidepressants has influenced this (see Chapter 7). As a result, in some cases, GPs are now prescribing a 'new' antidepressant and following the patient up themselves rather than, as was a common pattern a decade earlier, prescribing a tricyclic *and* a CPN!

Too close for comfort?

A year after our CPN department agreed to experiment with GP attachment, I began to wonder how comfortable our supposed closeness to primary care was proving. The CPN team was carved up – although it remains centrally based as part of the secondary care team – and CPNs were allocated to GP practices. The allocation was made according to something called 'contract value', which does not necessarily correlate with how much work each practice normally generates and, hence, there is an uneven distribution of work for different team members.

Early signs were not encouraging. Immediately upon making the switch to being 'GP-attached', we hit upon difficulties. To start with, a long-standing patient of mine refused to be either discharged or transferred to the CPN attached to the practice with which she was registered. A female patient with chronic anxiety problems, she angrily refused to see a female CPN and protested, in writing, to her own GP, psychologist and the Community Health Council. She made powerful arguments against the concept of GP-attachment.

I also had to discharge a woman with severe depression, who quietly accepted her fate. She did not wish to be transferred to the care of her would-be CPN because, after months struggling to describe her feelings to me, she could not face a fresh start.

We then faced some bizarre reversals. Patients I had only recently handed over to a new colleague were promptly handed back. Some expressed paranoid delusions about the CPN who had either stopped or started seeing them again. I wondered whether the stress of yet another change had exacerbated their illness. Two patients living in the same house ended up with two CPNs going in at different times of the day. This was a mixed blessing – less cost-effective but more individualised care.

One new referral said she would have preferred a woman but was so desperate for help she accepted me. Other new referrals included a man depressed over the break-up of his marriage and his ex-wife, who was also depressed for the same reason. I was unable to tell her that her ex-husband was also seeing me, although it clearly affected the counselling relationship. Previously, thanks to the close team-working of the CPNs, one CPN would have seen the woman, while a second CPN would have seen the man.

Next was a girl with depression and anorexia, whose brother I had previously seen in the same house a year earlier. I failed to realise this until I arrived at the house. She knew all about it and politely asked if she could be referred to a psychologist instead. Then there was the referral of a woman with an alcohol problem. She was ambivalent about seeing me because I had previously seen her mother, who eventually died of alcohol-related illness.

A woman who had been sexually abused as a child and raped as an adult was desperate for psychological help. She could not wait for a psychologist's appointment (the waiting list was several months) and, for the first time in my career, I was unable to offer her a female CPN because my colleagues were fully occupied with their own practice attachments. I was not used to practising in so inflexible a way, nor to feeling so powerless.

The referral rate of one practice (practice A) has not changed; it is still the largest referrer to the CPNs in our area but now these referrals are no longer shared among the team – they are all mine. The second (practice B) has begun to refer a trickle of new patients, still, quite rightly, favouring more severely ill patients. Practice C's one and only referral was made to me by the consultant psychiatrist rather than the GPs themselves.

There are stark differences in the relationship the practices have with me. Staff at practice A continue to be extremely friendly, informal, with no standing on ceremony. Practice B was keen on weekly meetings but the purpose of these was not clear; they seemed to have an important symbolic value. They also insisted on a 'message book', which does not seem to have significantly changed communication between us. I had always thought communication between us was excellent and was astounded when one doctor attacked me for our, reputedly, appalling lack of communication.

I mingle with the district nurses who tell me next time it is my turn to make the coffee, though it took me six months to work out whether or not I was allowed to make myself a cup. For a long time, I felt as if I was just visiting, and I doubt if I will ever become part of the furniture in the way that the district nurses are. As for practice C, I finally resorted to writing to them asking if they would consider inviting me to meet them.

None of the practices have made me feel as welcome as the one with which I was more loosely linked in the days before attachment. So, I still feel a little lost and lonely, more isolated from my colleagues, less appreciated by the GPs, perhaps a bit disowned by the trust that employs me.

Practice A has offered me the use of a consulting room which probably helps some patients, as well as the practice and myself. An invitation to practice B's Christmas party helped me feel better about GP-attachment but I have been waiting a year for a reply from practice C about my suggestion of a meeting.

I hope the system of GP-attachment will work better and feel more comfortable as time goes on. Meanwhile, I persevere, trying to do a full-time job for practice B, two full-time jobs for practice A and next to nothing for practice C.

Reflection

In the reflection preceding 'Too close for comfort?' I described the growing confidence and willingness of GPs to treat psychological illness without always involving the CPN. I suggested this was partly due to current government policy, such as the National Service Framework for Mental Health, but may also coincide with the availability of newer antidepressants. I get the impression that many GPs find 'new' antidepressants easy to prescribe and are happy to monitor the impact of these themselves without referral to secondary care. One GP I know used to often refer people for a 'bit of simple counselling' to accompany their antidepressant treatment. Presumably, it would not be worth employing a counsellor to do a 'bit of simple counselling' and the assumption is that 'simple counselling' (whatever that might be) is within the remit of a CPN.

If CPNs are supposed to be focusing on severe and enduring mental illness, and primary care is supposed to be dealing with more mental health problems without resorting to secondary care, there are a few choices to be made. One option is to employ CPNs directly in primary care. Another is to employ counsellors (and then to choose whether the counselling they provide should be 'simple' or more complex). Another option is to make full use of existing resources within primary care. Health visitors and practice nurses are a traditional part of the primary care landscape and could be used (and already are) to deal with mental health problems. In parts of the country, it is seen as more 'normal' for patients with schizophrenia to receive their depot neuroleptic injections from the practice nurse, rather than from a CPN. Post-natal depression is assessed and, to varying degrees, managed by health visitors.

My own experience of health visitors and practice nurses has been that there is tremendous variation in their levels of confidence and competence in the area of mental health care. Some health visitors seem very good at recognising when patients with depression or anxiety could benefit from seeing a CPN. What is often needed is somebody to argue for a change of antidepressant medication with the GP or to teach some basic anxiety management techniques. Sometimes, people simply need to see somebody outside their usual support networks, somebody who is concerned with them as a person and not just, for example, as a parent. One health visitor I knew had a great skill for helping patients disclose the fact they had been victims of abuse and then would refer them on to our service because she did not feel able to deal with this problem.

Practice nurses are an interesting professional group. In some ways, they are very much like CPNs. Patients often perceive them as highly skilled, competent and well respected, and frequently seem more satisfied by a consultation with the practice nurse than they would be with seeing the GP. Practice nurses often have additional expertise in the management of particular diseases, such as asthma. I have been surprised, however, through my attachment to primary care, to discover how circumscribed some practice nurses are by practice protocols and etiquette. For all their skill and expertise, practice nurses seem to enjoy far less autonomy – and particularly less autonomy from the medical profession – than do CPNs.

When I wrote about the role of the practice nurse in the management of depression I was interested, not only in the practicalities of this, but in how it would be perceived. I wanted to find out how practice nurses saw their role. I wanted to help patients receive the help they needed. I wanted practice nurses to feel more confident about dealing with depression and to know that there are a range of options. It seems to me that the essential thing is for health care workers to try to work in partnership. It is not about stepping on each other's toes or spoiling one another's patch. We should share knowledge, skills and resources to ensure people get the kind of help they need.

Managing depression in primary care – the role of the practice nurse

Clinical governance and depression in primary care

Clinical governance is more than just a 'buzz phrase'. With the publication of the government's White Paper, *The new NHS – modern, dependable*, clinical governance is set out as a framework for the way all healthcare should be delivered. Among its key principles are the day-to-day use of evidence-based practice, the systematic dissemination of good practice, ideas and innovations, and the gathering of high-quality data for monitoring clinical care. This article considers the impact clinical governance will have on the role of practice nurses with regard to an important area of mental health.

Of course, many practice nurses may already base their practice on available evidence; some are trying to disseminate their good practice and innovative ideas, others are involved in monitoring care through gathering data. Clinical governance's intention is that all this good practice will be drawn together in a systematic way to form part of each primary care organisation's clinical governance programme (Cook 1999).

One area where practice nurses may feel less confident about their practice is in their management of mental health problems. This could prove a large and worrying gap, given that, for example, about 5 per cent of the population are clinically depressed (Paykel and Priest 1992) and over 90 per cent of depressive episodes are managed in primary care (RCGP 1993). One practice nurse with whom I spoke admitted she had never had any training in recognising or treating depression. Another told me she was discouraged from offering 'talking time' to patients, while a third said she had offered a depressed patient support only to find it unmanageable when the patient sought her out, in a distressed state, at inconvenient times. Practice nurses, well placed as they are to help with this illness, clearly need to consider their role in the management of depression carefully.

Using effective interventions – physical, psychological and social

Clinical governance is about knowing which interventions are demonstrably effective, bringing these together systematically in the primary care organisation's programme and using them in practice. Therefore, we need to be clear about what is likely (and unlikely) to help the patient.

The evidence shows that the majority of depressed patients will respond to antidepressant medication or to talking treatments, or both (Blenkiron 1998). Antidepressants should not, however, be used in isolation or in every case and an individual's treatment plan should be negotiated with the patient to ensure optimal compliance and effectiveness (ibid.).

Practice nurses who take a more holistic approach to patients should appreciate that depression, like other forms of mental illness, is not a purely biophysical illness and it is therefore important to address the psychosocial aspects of the problem. The causes of an individual's depression can be as much to do with psychological factors (such as low self-esteem and lack of assertiveness) and with the person's social situation (e.g. factors such as relationship difficulties and unemployment). For these reasons, approaches such as cognitive behavioural therapy have been shown to be at least as effective as antidepressants in mild to moderate depression and can actually prevent recurrence of depression. While practice nurses could be trained to teach patients relaxation techniques and strategies for goal-setting and problem-solving, constraints on consultation time might be an important 'variable' in the success of this approach (ibid.).

Even if they lack the time or training to offer therapeutic interventions, well-informed practice nurses can at least educate, encourage and support depressed patients in the appropriate use of medication and guide patients towards other agencies that can help. These might include other professionals, like CPNs, mental health social workers, psychologists and psychiatrists, and also day care or support groups.

Recognising and managing depression

Recognising depressive illness is not always straightforward and if a practice nurse suspects a patient may be depressed, this should be taken seriously. Many patients value the opportunity to talk, in confidence, to somebody who they feel they can trust and who is non-judgemental. The nurse needs to check if the patient has been assessed by a professional skilled in the assessment and treatment of depression and to share her concerns about the patient with the GP, discussing whether antidepressants should be prescribed. In some cases, the patient may already be seeing a mental health worker. The practice nurse should liaise with others involved and consider her role in supporting the therapeutic process.

A major problem is compliance with medication. Patients may be dismissive of their own need for treatment or may feel hopeless about the prospects of getting better. They may also be experiencing troublesome side-effects. The practice nurse can help by reassuring patients that depression is an illness and, like other illnesses, can often be improved with medication. Most people with depression get better. All medication has side-effects and it is often a case of finding the medication that suits the person's symptoms best.

There are a few important points about antidepressants that practice nurses can reinforce with depressed patients. First, antidepressants are *not* addictive. Although sudden discontinuation has been identified as a problem, this can be managed by gradual tapering over a few weeks. Second, patients need to give their treatment a reasonable length of time to work (at least four weeks). Third, they should continue treatment for up to six months after recovery, in order to prevent a relapse (ibid.).

Conclusion

With further training, practice nurses could take a very proactive role in identifying depression, supporting recovery from the illness and preventing relapse. Such training is increasingly becoming available, through organisations like the Depression Care Training Centre. At the very least, with increased awareness of the facts about the illness – and the evidence of which treatments are effective – practice nurses could support other members of the primary and secondary care team in their treatment of depressed patients. We are only just beginning a debate about the respective roles of CPNs and practice nurses (Nolan *et al.* 1998). Clinical governance invites both groups of practitioners to become actively involved in the primary care organisation's programme. It is time we all liaised more closely to share good practice in the management of all mental health problems.

Reflection

Initiatives like the Lilly Schizophrenia Reintegration Awards bring about unexpected results. In Chapter 8, I described how my own project – the Music Workshop Project – had benefited from winning the award in 1998. Recognition is not a common feature of a CPN's job, so it is worth letting CPNs know more about such schemes.

The Schizophrenia Reintegration awards were set up in the mid-1990s as an international programme by Eli Lilly and Company and the World Psychiatric Association. The aim was to recognise outstanding achievement and innovation in reintegrating people with schizophrenia and related disorders back into society. Any individual or group involved in aspects of the reintegration process was eligible for entry. The winners were selected by an independent panel of leading experts in the field.

The awards originally covered three regions: Europe, Eastern Mediterranean and Latin America. However, in 1999 Lilly Psychiatry decided to introduce a UK competition specifically for projects in primary care, with a focus on multi-disciplinary working. The aim remains the same: to tackle the stigma of schizophrenia and promote better management of the illness. These annual awards are aimed at healthcare professionals who are based in, or have close links with, primary care. I was delighted and honoured to be asked to become one of the judges of the UK awards in 1999. I was also pleased that, while the themes of reintegration and innovation were retained, new emphasis was being placed on primary care and multi-disciplinary work.

Since the emergence of primary care groups in the UK there has been a need for GPs to start taking a more significant role in the management of people with mental health problems. Historically, schizophrenia is an area that GPs tend to refer on to secondary care. As a CPN based in secondary care but attached to GP practices, I am in a good position to overview the services offered generally to people with mental health problems by primary health care. Mostly, it seems, GPs have little contact with their patients with schizophrenia, trusting in the secondary mental health services to treat, maintain and reintegrate the patient. Sometimes a GP neglects to refer the patient to the appropriate secondary agencies when it would be helpful to obtain a more objective or more specialised intervention. In my own part of the country, the mental health services have implemented the Care Programme Approach (CPA), yet GPs seldom attend CPA reviews for their patients (perhaps because review meetings clash with peak surgery times). All too often, professionals in primary and secondary care end up blaming one another for the lack of communication.

By placing an emphasis on a multi-disciplinary, primary care approach for people with schizophrenia, the Reintegration Awards programme is sending out a crucial message. Practitioners in primary care need to ensure they are providing the best possible service to people with mental health problems, including those with severe and enduring illnesses, such as schizophrenia. This means offering well-informed, sensitive, comprehensive help within primary care, while also liaising when needed with secondary mental health care workers to obtain the very best treatment and care for patients. It involves not only greater two-way communication between primary and secondary care workers (and among health, social services and non-statutory organisations) but also an increased awareness and knowledge of the condition.

What is special about the project described in the article 'Putting innovation on the map' is that it is an example of general practice taking a particular interest in mentally ill people. Moreover, it is not just the mental health of these people that is being addressed but also their physical health. CPNs can often overlook the physical health of our patients in our concern for their psychological well-being. Good collaborative practice with primary care can ensure that both the physical and mental health needs of the community are met.

Putting innovation on the map

The Bronyffynnon Surgery

Denbigh, North Wales, is a market town a little off the beaten track. Despite countless childhood holidays and three years of student life in North Wales I never managed to visit the town, it being inland and south of the railway line that would take me from Chester towards the coastal resorts of Prestatyn and Rhyl. By car, the journey requires a detour off the A5 which runs implacably and impressively from Llangollen to Bangor and Holyhead. Denbigh nestles in the Vale of Clwyd, with a castle and a population half the size of its neighbouring Rhyl. Its most famous son was the explorer Sir Henry Morton Stanley (he of Livingstone fame). Not even the nineteenth-century travel writer George Borrow made it to Denbigh in his exploration of *Wild Wales*, despite marching from Chepstow to Holyhead. He did, however, learn from a fellow traveller that 'cheese made in the Vale of Clwyd fetches a penny a pound more than cheese made in any other valley' (Borrow 1977: 83).

It is, however, Denbigh's long association with mental illness that made it a fertile ground for a Reintegration Award winner. Denbigh was the site of the former North Wales Hospital which was one of the largest mental hospitals in Wales prior to its closure in the 1980s. The hospital served a catchment area covering north and mid Wales, parts of Cheshire and Merseyside. Upon closure, most of its residents were discharged into the local community, either into residential care homes or to live independently, supported by the community mental health services. In common with other large psychiatric institutions, many of its residents had been in the hospital so long they were not capable of independent living. This demand for residential care led to several private care homes being founded in the region.

Swelling this population is a large independent-sector mental health rehabilitation unit based at a former sanatorium about five miles from Denbigh. This provides specialist care for 50 people with severe mental health problems who need institutional care as a stepping stone towards reintegration in the community. Clients come from all over the UK, referred by social services departments whose own local mental health care establishments are unable to cope with their particular problems.

Bronyffynnon, the main local general practice, consequently has a large number of patients with chronic mental illness on its list. While the accepted incidence of schizophrenia in the UK is one per cent, some ten per cent of patients registered with the Bronyffynnon practice have a severe mental illness. In one typical three-month period, the practice issued approximately 1,650 prescriptions for antipsychotic medication, of which 363 were for the new generation of drugs, such as risperidone and olanzapine – an unusually high usage for a GP surgery. As a result, all members of the primary care team have developed a greater degree of expertise in mental health care than that found in most practices.

1999 – focusing on primary care

Bronyffynnon was winner of the 1999 Lilly Schizophrenia Reintegration Award, which, in that year, had decided to focus specifically on projects in primary care that involved multi-disciplinary working. The aim of the awards remains that of destigmatising schizophrenia and achieving better management of the illness. However, since the emergence of primary care groups in the UK there has been a need for GPs to start taking a more significant role in the management of people with mental health problems. The winning project was an annual health screening programme for people on the practice register with chronic mental health problems. The service currently screens about 120 patients with acute and chronic mental health problems living in residential care and registered as patients with the practice. The screening includes the offer of a physical examination, assessment of the patient's current psychological status, discussion of any problems that the patient or their carers may raise and arranging any monitoring investigations that may be indicated.

Andrew Heaton, one of the four GPs involved in the Bronyffynnon project, describes the rationale for the screening process: 'It's an unfortunate fact that patients with mental illness tend to receive very cursory treatment from the NHS, often because they are difficult to manage, are poor historians and default readily from follow-up'. Community mental health services, he argues, understandably concentrate on their clients' mental health problems and many people with mental health problems rarely present to their GPs with a physical problem or even recognise that they do, in fact, have a physical problem. Indeed, many are not even registered with a GP. It is this gap in holistic care that inspired the screening initiative.

Physical health of mentally ill people

It has been recognised that severely mentally ill people, perhaps because they may tend to smoke heavily, follow a less healthy lifestyle in terms of exercise and diet and present later with physical illness, often receiving sub-optimal treatment. It is now almost a decade since the *Health of the Nation* government White Paper highlighted the fact that mentally ill people have extremely high death rates from common physical illnesses, like heart disease and cancers (Department of Health 1992). Outcomes of the Bronyffynnon screening process include diagnoses of ischaemic heart disease and cancer, which might otherwise have gone untreated, along with the identification of thyroid disease, hypertension and respiratory problems. Blood tests are also carried out to monitor drugs, such as lithium, carbamazepine, phenytoin, clozapine and risperidone, to ensure they are not adversely affecting patients' thyroid or liver function. The screening also provides the opportunity to review each patient's current immunisation status. As a result, a campaign to update all polio immunisations has been launched to run alongside the annual influenza vaccination programme. Screening has also picked up on deficiencies in many patients' hepatitis B immunisation status.

Originally intended to be a stand-alone service, the screening programme has now become an established part of surgery routine at Bronyffynnon. The actual screening examination takes about thirty minutes and is carried out at a clinic provided by the local Denbigh Infirmary community hospital, in time allocated from normal surgery commitments. However, any follow-up referrals and reviews have to be squeezed into the routine surgery appointments system. A sign of the practice's commitment to the programme is that locum GPs are used when necessary to provide cover for the GPs while they do the screening.

Out-patient services manager Fiona Turner says the award has made an important difference to the programme:

> Since winning the award the doctors have been able to increase their time so they now come twice a week to do the screening. We book just four patients at a time, and the patients and their carers appreciate the extra time and not having to wait.

She also believes the screening programme has helped promote better understanding and acceptance of mentally ill people in the community and among nurses and doctors in the area: 'The fact that they see mentally ill people regularly means it now doesn't bother people. It's accepted that they need the same treatment as others.'

Annual screening is not new. Arguably, it is a sad indictment of our health care system that a simple screening programme is singled out for an innovation award. Be that as it may, it is undoubtedly innovative to pay attention, systematically and in equal measure, to the physical, as well as the psychological, needs of so disadvantaged and vulnerable a group of people. As Cliff Prior, chief executive of the National Schizophrenia Fellowship (co-sponsor of the Award), said of Bronyffynnon's initiative:

> It is a simple and straightforward project, but one of enormous importance to people with severe mental illness. The fact that it has been done with very limited resources within a busy GP practice is very positive in that it is much more likely to be replicable around the country.

While it may be over-optimistic to expect every primary care team to instigate a similar screening programme, it is perhaps not too much to expect all those working in primary care to learn lessons from Bronyffynnon. First, the physical health needs of the mentally ill should not be neglected. Second, the treatment of illnesses such as schizophrenia needs to be optimised by regular systematic review, screening, monitoring for side-effects, tolerance and compliance, and making changes accordingly. Third, primary care should share with secondary care responsibility for mental health. This means striking a balance between extremes. At one extreme is the arrogant belief that primary care can single-handedly manage all the problems. At the other is the belief that mentally ill people should be hurriedly referred on to secondary care where all their needs will be met. Both of these are myths.

Primary care can and should provide considerable help to mentally ill people, so long as practitioners in all disciplines are better informed about new and existing treatments. Secondary care needs to liaise closely with primary care to ensure that physical health needs are being addressed. These are some of the lessons to be learnt from Bronyffynnon. People working in the field of mental health should not be afraid to innovate and it is worth noting that the good work of reintegration often takes place initially in the absence of extra recognition or resources. Happily, initiatives like the Lilly Schizophrenia Reintegration Awards exist to provide something of both.

10 We are family
Family interventions

Reflection

When I first became a CPN, I was approached by the co-ordinators of various services. The psychologist leading the Parasuicide Team wondered if I would be interested in becoming a parasuicide counsellor. The co-ordinator of Anxiety Management Groups thought I might like to help to run the next anxiety management group. There seemed to be a number of opportunities to diversify beyond the traditional one-to-one home visits that formed the bread and butter work of a CPN. One of these 'extra-curricular activities' that captured my imagination was something called the Family Therapy Interest Group. This group was really no more than its name implied – a group of people who had an interest in family therapy.

My interest in family work began as a student nurse when I attended a day workshop organised by a family therapist from Cardiff. I had read a few articles and one or two books but had never had any formal training in working with families. However, one of the attractions of the CPN's job is the contact we have with families by going into people's homes. I was interested in the relationship between community psychiatric nursing, our routine contact with families and the concept of family therapy as a specialist intervention. I examined this in the article 'Family therapy – exploring the role of the CPN'. The article was written from the point of view of a CPN who has an interest (but no specialist training) in family therapy. It now reads as a rather old-fashioned overview of classical models of family therapy but it is interesting to compare the concepts described here with the later descriptions of family interventions. For instance, few proponents of family interventions in psychosis would suggest stopping medication while the family therapy takes place. This kind of purism would be seen as at best precious and at worst dangerous.

Chapter 10, then, begins with a discussion about family therapy in general. It then moves on, more specifically, to the theory behind psychoeducational interventions with the families of people with schizophrenia. In many ways, these family interventions have very little to do with the kinds of family therapy described in the first article here. Finally, it describes attempts to put the theory of psychoeducational interventions into practice, in two case studies.

Family therapy – exploring the role of the CPN

Family therapy is often listed as one of a range of areas within which the CPN might specialise. For example, Simmons and Brooker (1986) wrote of the 'growing expertise among mental health professionals in non-drug therapies, including counselling, behaviour therapy, family therapy, social skills training'. They suggested that 'Having carried out a full assessment, the CPN may decide to offer one of a range of different types of therapy' . . . [including] . . . 'family meetings or therapy' (ibid.).

While it might be assumed that all CPNs are capable of offering a range of interventions, no single CPN can be expected to have developed an expertise in every area. It would be misleading to suggest that, if family therapy is seen as the treatment of choice, then that indeed is what the CPN will offer. CPNs may not feel qualified to offer family therapy themselves and there may not be a family therapy service locally to which clients can be referred. Simmons and Brooker (1986) acknowledge that:

> Various factors affect the type of therapy or care provided by CPNs for their clients. The most important of these is, of course, the type of problems identified by the client, the family and the CPN. However, CPNs will also select different methods depending on their own interests, philosophies of mental health and illness, and the skills they possess.
>
> (ibid.)

Like most, if not all, psychological treatments, family therapy is surrounded by debate. What is it? When is it appropriate? Who should implement it? In which setting should it be implemented? Is specialised training required? If so, how will this be validated?

Family therapy seems to encompass a spectrum of approaches. In one sense, the term is used to describe the involvement and support of family members in the care of an individual. In another, it is a specific psychological therapy practised by specialised family therapists in a controlled and structured way. CPNs must examine their understanding of the concept so they can work collaboratively with patients and families. The assumption of this article is that even those CPNs who have no special interest in the subject must clarify their own position if they are to avoid colluding against the patient.

The great uncertainty about family therapy is reflected in the literature. Clayton (1989) points out, quizzically, 'Everyone knows about family therapy, but who actually practises it?' Clayton's view of field social workers applies equally to CPNs:

> [They] believe family therapy to be effective and know something about the techniques used. But most have gained this knowledge from reading, speaking to someone or by joining one of the various groups set up to discuss the merits of family therapy and offer support to practitioners.

Rarely does one come across fellow professionals in the field who are actually practising.

(Clayton 1989)

In stark contrast to Simmons and Brooker's idealised image of CPNs who can, with unquestioned credibility, turn their hand to family therapy, Sheehy (1990) described the suspicion surrounding nurses' claims to be able to offer family therapy:

> Nurses' relationships with other disciplines in the health service have been contentious at times when management structures or fantasies about each other's abilities cloud or damage working relationships. In mental health . . . questions about what nurses can or cannot do, regardless of their reality, may lead nurses to feel they have to prove themselves in particular therapeutic settings . . . it had been hinted (nurses felt) . . . that nurses were not qualified to practise certain therapies alone.

(Sheehy 1990: 8)

Walrond-Skinner (1976), cited in Carr *et al.* (1980), stated that: 'Family therapy can be defined as the psychotherapeutic treatment of a natural social system'. It is unclear whether this means formal psychotherapy sessions with a family or, more generally, working in a psychotherapeutic way with the family. However, the use of the term 'treatment' might imply a more formal, structured approach.

Walrond-Skinner's definition (1976) can be contrasted with that of McDonald (1987), who wrote:

> Family therapy is the involvement of the entire family in the treatment process, based on the understanding that a particular symptom or group of symptoms, although perhaps exhibited by only one family member, has emerged because of underlying tensions in the family.

(McDonald 1987: 46)

It might be assumed that, if family therapy is simply involving the family therapeutically in the process of treating the client, then all CPNs are engaged in family therapy. Encouraging as this belief might seem, it is here that a historical complication arises. The family has historically only been of interest to the CPN in so far as it is the family of the patient. Thus, CPNs have tended to work either with the patient in isolation or with the family as an adjunct to that patient. Rarely has the family itself been viewed as the 'patient'.

Much of the literature on community psychiatric nursing refers to the families of clients as 'carers'. This may reflect the large proportion of elderly mentally ill clients and of long-term severely mentally ill clients with which community psychiatric nursing has traditionally concerned itself. In reviewing the literature, Pollock (1989) noted that:

Community psychiatric nursing contact is also considered beneficial to the carers who, it is argued, receive support and also relief at the earliest opportunity. The discussion . . . suggests that the 'family' (especially female kin) are expected to look after sick members.

(ibid.)

Pollock (1989) went on to examine to what extent supporting the 'carers' affected the work of CPNs. She identified two trains of thought as regards the family and the work of the CPN. The first of these is that changing a client's family situation is really beyond the scope of a CPN's work. The second is that the CPN should take an active role with the family, looking for stresses within the family and taking steps to remedy these. The two approaches can be broadly categorised as, respectively, the medical model and the social model of care.

In Pollock's analysis, families or carers are seen as largely irrelevant (following the medical model) or else as a suitable area of concern for CPNs (following the social model) due to the stresses of caring. The implication behind supporting carers under stress is that, first, they may fall victim to mental illness themselves and, second, that their stress may exacerbate the illness of the identified client. Nowhere, however, does Pollock make the leap into a more radical social model in which families can be seen negatively as part of the illness or problem, or positively as part of the treatment or solution.

It is making explicit the family's direct relationship to mental illness that propels community psychiatric nursing into the arena of family therapy. In many ways, references to 'supporting the family' and, more tritely, 'caring for the carers', take us far from the perspectives that enable family therapy to take place.

Based on McDonald's (1987) definition, it was suggested that family therapy might be simply an approach that can inform much of the CPNs' work with individual clients. What, then, of the interpretation of family therapy more formally, as a kind of psychotherapy with the family? The word 'psychotherapy' raises controversies similar to those surrounding family therapy. CPNs may be happier claiming to be able to offer counselling than to say they practise psychotherapy (Cooper 1987). In the light of this, it is interesting to note the confidence of the social workers attempting family therapy (Clayton 1989) compared with the self-doubt of the CPNs who set up and ran a family therapy clinic (Sheehy 1990).

A further complication is that family therapy is not a single theory or a single package of skills and techniques. There are many theories and a corresponding variety of styles of intervention. McMahon (1990), for instance, suggested that family therapists tend to belong to one of three subgroups, which he categorised as 'the conductors', 'the reactor-analysts' and the 'systems purists' (see Table 10.1). Even this, according to McMahon, is merely a broad framework within which therapists develop their own styles.

Table 10.1 Three subgroups of family therapists (adapted from McMahon (1990))

1. *The conductors* see their role as being to re-educate the family in more healthy and creative attitudes. These therapists will openly confront the pathological functioning of the family. This group includes such workers as Ackerman, Virginia Satir and Salvador Minuchin.
2. *The reactor-analysts* use their own emotional response (counter-transference) as a means of understanding and changing the family pathology, according to psychoanalytic precepts.
3. *The systems purists*, such as Jay Haley, endeavour to change the ground rules of relationships within the family to promote constructive change.

McDonald sees the focus of all family therapy as the treatment of the family as the primary unit, 'rather than any individual member who has been defined as "patient" or "identified patient" (IP)' (1987: 46). He recommended that, if possible, other forms of psychiatric treatment of the IP should be discontinued for the duration of the family therapy. Adhering to this may well bring the CPN into conflict with medical colleagues and test the limits of the CPN's credibility within the multi-disciplinary team.

McDonald sees the goals of family therapy as the reduction of conflict and anxiety, the promotion of awareness of each other's needs, the development of appropriate role relationships and the promotion of health. However, drawing on Minuchin (1974), McDonald (1987) stated that, above all, family therapy is indicated for 'dysfunctional families'. Minuchin (1974) identified a number of characteristics, the absence of which renders a family dysfunctional. These include such things as 'appropriate emotional distance', 'the encouragement of differences' and 'age appropriateness'. Alternatively, Cooper (1987) based his family therapy intervention on family systems theory. He saw family therapy as having five basic tenets (see Table 10.2).

Table 10.2 Cooper's five basic tenets of family therapy intervention (adapted from Cooper (1987))

1. The family is more than a collection of individuals, the whole is greater than the sum of its parts.
2. Families have repeating interaction patterns that regulate members' behaviour. (Implicit rules are often not spoken and there may be family rituals. Analysis of these patterns of interaction is the chief assessment tool.)
3. Individuals' symptoms may serve a functional need within the family.
4. The ability to adapt, for example, to children growing up, is the hallmark of a healthy family.
5. Family members share joint responsibility for their problems, there are no victims and victimisers.

It is difficult to trace any clear historical development of family therapy in relation to community psychiatric nursing. It is apparent, however, that those articles on family therapy that have been published in the nursing press are often written by CPNs. It is also interesting to note the sweeping statements in bold print that have been used to introduce such articles. For example, McDonald wrote: 'Psychiatric nurses with their interpersonal skills and understanding of behavioural techniques are ideally suited to working with families' (1987: 46). Cooper was of a similar opinion: 'Family therapy is gaining increasing acceptance among psychiatric nurses' (1987: 62). While both these comments may be true, they perhaps give a false impression of the extent to which family therapy is used by psychiatric nurses. Nonetheless, it would seem that, where family therapy is being used by nurses, those nurses are often CPNs.

Family therapy has begun to develop beyond a special interest of a number of generic CPNs into an area of specialisation. Resistance to this trend might be expected, particularly where a family approach conflicts with the medical model, for instance, where it recommends the suspension of other treatments for the duration of the family therapy. Apart from the medical model, conflict is also possible with less radical versions of the social model, wherein other members are seen as carers of the identified patient. The prevalence of this approach, held dear by those CPNs who have tried to espouse a social model over and above the medical model, may, ironically, be so great a force as to obstruct the widespread application of family therapy by CPNs. Perhaps what is needed is a view of family therapy that takes in the whole spectrum of definitions.

In some cases, it will be appropriate to use a rigorous, highly structured and controlled form of family therapy, requiring specific techniques and skills practised by CPNs who at the least have some specialist training even if they are not being employed specifically as family therapists. In other cases, a looser approach will be called for, wherein the patient is treated within the family context, using some of the insights of family therapy, without offering a course of family treatment as such. In yet other cases, it may be enough to work with the 'identified patient' as if there were no family. Having gained some awareness of family therapy, however, it would seem unlikely, if not impossible, that CPNs' practice could fail to be informed by this controversial yet compelling approach.

Reflection

Family interventions can be effective in the management of schizophrenia. However, there are many obstacles to the use of the techniques, both organisational and ideological. There are also practical problems and ethical dilemmas. The article 'The case for using family interventions in the management of schizophrenia' argues that solutions to these obstacles are at hand.

Family intervention involves supportive, educational and therapeutic interaction with the families of people with schizophrenia, in order to decrease stress within the family unit and reduce the risk of relapse. It is an adjunct, rather than an alternative, to drug treatment. Strategies include a combination of educating family members about schizophrenia and training in problem-solving. Changing attitudes and behaviour among relatives and helping families manage stress are also involved. Some detractors have taken delight, recently, in suggesting that the evidence for family interventions is less and less compelling. Be that as it may, the evidence continues to suggest the importance of family interventions in reducing relapse rates. Moreover, recent policy developments support the promotion of family-sensitive services. There are, therefore, what might be described as both 'hard' and 'soft' arguments for family interventions. That is, there are scientific and human reasons why we should work together with families.

The case for using family interventions in the management of schizophrenia

Family interventions have been found to be effective as an adjunct to drug therapy in the management of schizophrenia. A meta-analysis of research findings was carried out by the Cochrane Schizophrenia Group, which set out to estimate the effectiveness of family psychosocial interventions in community settings for the care of those with schizophrenia-like conditions (Mari *et al.* 1997). Their review found that family intervention for people with schizophrenia reduced the rate of relapse at 12, 18 and 24 months. It also reduced hospital admission rates at both one year and over the period of 13–18 months and helped improve compliance with medication. Subsequent updates by the Cochrane Schizophrenia Group, though less compelling, continue to show that family intervention decreases the risk of relapse.

Naturally, with reductions in rates of relapse and hospitalisation, and with improved compliance with medication, it would seem that psychosocial interventions might lead to a reduction in overall costs of treatment. This was certainly suggested by those studies in the review that paid attention to economic analyses (ibid.). Analyses of cost in health care are complex but reductions in hospitalisation are likely to correlate with significant savings.

What remains unclear from the Cochrane Review is which particular aspects of family intervention were responsible for the observed reduction in relapse rates for schizophrenia. Droogan and Brannigan suggest that 'the change in relapse and hospitalisation rates may, for example, be due to the increased level of contact people with schizophrenia receive from health care professionals who engage in psychosocial interventions' (Droogan and Brannigan 1997: 47). Consideration needs to be given, then, to what constitutes family intervention in order for it to be effective. Since the emphasis in the research is on schizophrenia, its effectiveness in other psychoses also needs further exploration.

Defining family intervention

Terminology can add to the confusion when discussing family intervention. First, the term 'family therapy' – though a convenient 'catch-all' for clinicians – is generally avoided in much of the relevant literature because it seems to denote either systemic or psychodynamic styles of family work. The exception to this is where 'family therapy' is predicated by the word 'behavioural' (Falloon *et al.* 1996). After avoiding 'family therapy', the preferred terminology would seem to be 'psychoeducational interventions', which, according to Fadden, should encompass the terms 'psychosocial', 'psychoeducational and family interventions', and 'family management approaches' (Fadden 1998).

Fadden has provided an indispensable definition of psychoeducational interventions: 'those interventions where the patient and family members are seen together, where there is a skills acquisition component in addition to a didactic element and where the primary aim is reduction of relapse in the patient' (ibid.). Fadden distinguishes 'psychoeducational interventions' from what she terms 'interventions with relatives', which usually refers to 'interventions directed at relatives (excluding the patient) and where the primary focus is on the needs of the family members rather than on the prevention of relapse in the patient' (ibid.).

The Cochrane Review took a fairly broad view of family intervention. The interventions included in the review were any psychological interventions with relatives of people with schizophrenia that required more than five sessions (Mari *et al.* 1997). Falloon, reviewing 22 controlled studies since 1980, seemed to advocate a 'mixed economy' of interventions: 'The approaches can be delivered in single family groups, multiple family groups, separate groups of relatives and patients, and in groups of residents in non-family households' (Falloon 1998). The prerequisite to this eclecticism and flexibility, however, was that the family interventions should be long term, cognitive – behavioural in orientation and integrated with optimal drug and case management (ibid.).

Fourteen features of psychosocial intervention

Fadden has identified 14 features that are common to successful psychosocial interventions in schizophrenia (Fadden 1998), which are worth listing in full here (see Table 10.3).

Fadden's 14 features would seem to concur with Falloon's review of successful interventions (Falloon 1998). Both stress the importance of optimal medication alongside any family work and a behavioural or cognitive–behavioural orientation. The only types of approach that have been shown to be effective are those that are psychoeducational in nature. Psychodynamic family interventions (where, for example, painful unconscious feelings are brought to the surface to be experienced and understood) have been shown to

Table 10.3 Fadden's 14 features of successful psychosocial intervention in
schizophrenia (adapted from Fadden (1998))

1. The acceptance of a vulnerability–stress model of schizophrenia.
2. The person with schizophrenia is maintained on medication.
3. Intervention begins during, or soon after, an acute episode when family motivation is high.
4. The development of a positive working alliance between family and therapist.
5. Patient and family are seen together for at least some of the intervention sessions.
6. Some, if not all, of the intervention sessions are conducted in the family home.
7. An emphasis on family education and provision of information about the disorder in order to enhance understanding.
8. A behavioural or cognitive–behavioural orientation with an emphasis on practical day-to-day issues.
9. The enhancement of family problem-solving skills.
10. Changes in communication patterns in the family, resulting in greater clarity of expression and less emotive exchanges between family members.
11. The reduction of unpleasant family atmosphere because of reduced stress and enhanced coping strategies.
12. The maintenance of realistic expectations for the patient and for other family members.
13. The encouragement of interests outside the family for all family members through a process of goal-setting, expansion of social networks or participation in family group or support meetings.
14. Interventions are maintained over a period of time with follow-up, or take place in the context of ongoing service.

be ineffective (Kottgen *et al.* 1984; McFarlane 1994). Similarly, a short-term family counselling approach seems to have failed (Vaughan *et al.* 1992).

Both Fadden and Falloon stress that the psychoeducational intervention should be long term and both allude to the work taking place in the context of ongoing service provision and optimal case management. Although Falloon seems to be recommending a combination of psychoeducational interventions involving the patient and interventions with relatives *excluding* the patient, Fadden's 14 features seem to favour the former over the latter, with their emphasis on seeing the patient together with the family and preferably in the family's own home.

Family interventions in other psychoses

If psychoeducational interventions have been shown to be effective in the management of schizophrenia, what then of other psychoses? The Cochrane Review included patients with a standardised diagnosis of schizophrenia and/or schizo-affective disorder (Mari *et al.* 1997). This is noteworthy since the few studies that have attempted to apply family intervention in disorders other than schizophrenia have focused attention on an affective psychosis, namely bipolar disorder.

Although the findings are not so overwhelmingly persuasive as the research into schizophrenia, there is enough (Goldstein and Miklowitz 1994; Glick *et al.* 1994; Clarkin *et al.* 1990; Anderson *et al.* 1986) to suggest that family interventions are indeed effective in the management of at least one other type of psychosis. More research is needed to establish whether people with bipolar illness stand to gain as much from family interventions as people with schizophrenia. Equally, it would be premature to assume family interventions are effective in all types of psychotic illness, although it would be surprising if, given the weight of evidence, these interventions proved to be completely unhelpful in, say, psychotic depression or puerperal psychosis.

Implementation

While, as has been shown, there is good evidence for the effectiveness of family interventions, there is a parallel body of evidence suggesting that implementation is fraught with difficulties. Backer and colleagues indicate that the mere dissemination of information about innovative approaches does not necessarily guarantee that they will be adopted in clinical practice (Backer *et al.* 1986). There are a number of obstacles to implementation. These may include the attitude of staff if the approach conflicts with established concepts and practices, and organisational barriers such as the wide range of other interests and motivations found in the organisation. One particular factor may be conflicting pressures on the service from outside sources. This is very evident, for example, in the case of CPNs who, under the system of GP fundholding, found themselves increasingly pressurised into focusing on primary care priorities which, typically, include an emphasis on individual patients rather than families and an emphasis on mental health problems other than schizophrenia (Gillam 1994, 1998).

Other research has supported the view that implementation of family psychoeducational interventions is hampered by conflicts with the theoretical training of many clinicians. McFarlane suggests other obstacles include the complexity of an approach and the fact that its outcomes emerge in the long term (McFarlane 1994). Of course, the length of time needed for outcomes to emerge is relative. It can be hard convincing a psychiatrist whose patient has relapsed and been re-admitted after six months of family interventions that these treatments do indeed reduce the rate of relapse at 12, 18 and 24 months, and reduce admission rates at one year and over the period of 13–18 months (Mari *et al.* 1997). Six months must be regarded as 'early days' in the intervention but this may be hard to 'sell' to doctors used to drugs taking effect within weeks if not days, and to nurse managers and social work managers who see their staff 'tied up' for several hours a week with one family, only to see that patient back on the ward.

Obstacles to intervention can be said to be either organisational or ideological, although there is considerable overlap. Organisational obstacles might include staff resistance to change, inflexibility of working practice and

competing service priorities. Ideological obstacles are, perhaps, more subjective and individualised, and might include clinicians' confidence and
competence in working with families or groups in contrast to the more usual
individualised approach. This may be based on ingrained professional training, which neglects family and group approaches to treatment.

Confidentiality

One particular stumbling block seems to be the issue of confidentiality, which
has traditionally led to a reluctance to discuss the identified patient's problems with family members. This ethical dilemma has been considered by
Szmukler and Bloch who acknowledge that 'the crucial role of carers in
making "community care" possible is increasingly recognised, carrying with
it a right to respect their needs', but that 'achieving optimal collaboration
with the family is often beset with difficulties of an ethical nature, especially
revolving around confidentiality, and its potential breach' (Szmukler and
Bloch 1997: 401).

Furlong and Leggatt concur that:

> Clinicians in all First World communities confront a dilemma in relation
> to confidentiality. What is new, or at least becoming clearer, is the premise
> that clinicians should relate to the families of the mentally ill in a manner
> that is more sensitive than was previously expected.
>
> (Furlong and Leggatt 1996: 614)

They go on to argue that, although this idea may have become more accepted:

> It is often less than clear to clinicians how a balance can be found
> between the rights and interests of patients and the needs and responsi-
> bilities of carers. Clinicians seek to respect the right of patients to
> self-determination and to develop relationships with patients charac-
> terised by trust within which greater patient autonomy can develop.
> Clinicians also perceive that confidentiality is a legal right for patients.
> Yet, clinicians do wish to respect the position of carers whom they
> increasingly recognise as undertaking significant responsibilities and
> enduring persistent burden.
>
> (Furlong and Leggatt 1996: 614–15)

This dilemma may well be one of the obstacles to mental health workers
implementing family interventions. The whole area is perceived as a minefield
of ethical problems, which could lead to accusations of professional miscon-
duct or even litigation. If clinicians feel they lack the support of their
organisation they might understandably feel it is wiser to steer clear of family
interventions. Yet, in the light of the evidence, clinicians are faced with
another moral dilemma. Fadden has argued that, given the fact that family

interventions in schizophrenia have been shown to be effective, that they are not being offered routinely to sufferers of schizophrenia and their families is 'morally inexcusable' (Fadden 1997: 610). Recent policy developments, such as the National Service Framework for Mental Health, in their insistence on the rights of carers and families to receive appropriate support, reinforce this cultural shift.

If clinicians, and service planners and providers, cannot in all conscience withhold such an effective treatment for such a severe illness then they must grasp the nettle and find new ways of dealing with ethical dilemmas as they arise. It is also incumbent on service managers to ensure that clinicians are sufficiently prepared for family interventions (through adequate training) and sufficiently supported (through adequate supervision).

Partnership between clinicians and families

Before considering ways of training and supervising clinicians, it is worth revisiting the ethical arguments posed earlier. This is not only because clinicians will need practical solutions but because such a discussion throws light on what has been termed in this article 'ideological obstacles'. Furlong and Leggatt describe how, between the late 1980s and the late 1990s, there have been significant developments in how mental health professionals perceive the relatives of those with mental illness. 'The current literature argues that these clinicians should regard families as "allies" and "partners" in treatment and rehabilitation.' This, they believe, is partly due to the process of deinstitutionalisation, with more patients living with their relatives, but is 'also likely to be the result of more enlightened and less blaming attitudes towards the families of the mentally ill' (Furlong and Leggatt 1996: 615).

The shift towards a commitment to partnership between clinicians and families is seen as a significant development, away from past relationships influenced by psychoanalytic and anti-psychiatry ideas. Research into 'expressed emotion' – the concept that the emotional climate of the patient's home, the levels of criticism, hostility and involvement of the family having an impact on the illness – brought a more scientific perspective (Brown *et al.* 1972). Furlong and Leggatt, however, noted that even research into expressed emotion (or 'EE') can be misinterpreted by clinicians and be used as a rationale for blaming families for patient relapse if not aetiology: if patients returning to 'high EE' families tend to relapse, it follows that these families need to be conscripted into educational programmes in order for the families to become 'better environments' for patients (Furlong and Leggatt 1996).

It is imperative that Fadden's 14 features, which are common to successful psychosocial interventions in schizophrenia, are kept in mind. Particular emphasis must be given to three of these features. First, the development of a positive working alliance between family and therapist. If the therapist is to maintain a positive attitude, arguments about 'high EE' are best avoided. Secondly, the reduction of unpleasant family atmosphere because of reduced stress and enhanced coping strategies. Highlighting examples of 'high EE' runs the risk of reinforcing the unpleasant atmosphere while doing little to reduce the stress. Thirdly, a behavioural or cognitive–behavioural orientation with an emphasis on practical day-to-day issues is recommended precisely because this lends itself to reinforcing positive behaviour and positive thinking rather than reinforcing negative feelings.

Training and supervision

Leff *et al.* (1982) recommended systematic training in family interventions for professional mental health staff. The importance of specific training in family intervention techniques has been shown in more recent studies, which indicate that effective results are not produced in the absence of specialised training in applying the interventions (Vaughan *et al.* 1992; McCreadie *et al.* 1991). Both these studies identify lack of training as a major reason for lack of success in implementation. In reviewing family intervention studies, Fadden identified staff training and supervision as 'the most essential element which determined whether or not interventions were successful' (Fadden 1998). It is noteworthy that Fadden groups 'training and supervision' together as '*one* essential element', implying that – like the old song about love and marriage – you cannot have one without the other!

This is borne out by Brennan and Gamble's (1997) study of mental health nurses' training in family interventions. They recommend that training should be provided at every level and that training should be multi-disciplinary. They see supervision as an important means of reducing the isolation of those trained:

> To reduce the likelihood of family workers becoming isolated, post-course supervision should be incorporated into clinical areas. This would address problems such as not seeing progress, and lacking confidence in their general family work skills, as well as maintaining clinical competence.
>
> (Brennan and Gamble 1997: 15)

Training, it would seem, is only the beginning of the process but many of the organisational and ideological obstacles can be overcome by a continuing programme of initial training and ongoing supervision.

The number of therapists trained in any given service area is obviously a key factor in implementation. This is underlined by a study by Kavanagh *et al.* (1988),which reported that, of 160 therapists trained, only 44 took part in the treatment trial, and 57 per cent of the study participants were seen by six therapists. It used to be said that general nursing students were recruited in excessively high numbers to allow for an excessive drop-out rate. There is a feeling that family therapy trainees are also a little like 'cannon-fodder' – many more need to be trained so that we are, at least, left with a few. This is a difficult argument to put convincingly to health and social service managers (especially in this age of efficiency and value for money).

Managers might prefer it if training were targeted on those therapists working in the community, since Fadden (1997) argued that a community location (normally the families' own homes) had a positive influence on uptake of interventions. Arguably, though, clinicians working in in-patient units need at least an understanding of the approach if the culture of local mental health services is to be conducive to those carrying out family interventions.

Conclusion

It is clear that training and supervision are keystones in the successful implementation of family interventions. An understanding of the effectiveness of family interventions urgently needs to become part of every mental health professional's basic training. If sufficient numbers of clinicians are then trained in its techniques, a 'critical mass' will emerge, offering a positive benefit to families and improving the outlook for people with schizophrenia in our society.

Reflection

The term 'family intervention' is a catch-all used to describe a wide range of work with the families of people with schizophrenia. The following two case studies describe the use specifically of Behavioural Family Therapy (BFT), an approach taught in the West Midlands-based Meriden family interventions training programme, which I undertook. The Meriden programme is a regional cascade training programme established in 1997 under the auspices of the Evidence-supported Medicine Union (EMU). It is led by psychologist Gráinne Fadden who trained and supervised two BFT trainers from each mental health trust in the region, so that they could, in turn, train other mental health workers in their trusts to offer the approach to families. The training is evaluated and monitored at regional level. Ongoing supervision of both the training and the clinical practice has been provided to the trainers, while the trainers provide ongoing clinical supervision to the practitioners they have trained within our own trusts. The Meriden programme has attracted interest nationally and internationally, and has advised and, in some cases, conducted training programmes in family interventions abroad.

I always had the feeling that CPNs should address the needs of families (and particularly families where there were people with severe and enduring mental illness). I was not convinced, however, that any of the approaches described in 'Family therapy – exploring the role of the CPN' would be of much practical help. When I was introduced to psychoeducational family interventions, I realised that here was a powerful tool with which to help families. It had credibility, in that it was 'evidence-based', and it targeted people with psychosis. While 'The case for using family interventions in the management of schizophrenia' set out the theoretical arguments for this approach, this final section of the book closes with two examples of putting this theory into practice.

Two case studies of psychoeducational family interventions

Case study one: Listening to what Simon says

Simon

Simon (all names have been changed to protect the family's identity) was 26 when I first met him, and was diagnosed with a psychotic illness. He apparently first became ill in his early twenties, initially with what was thought to be a depressive illness. He was prescribed an antidepressant and referred to a CPN who suspected that he might have a psychosis. When he was assessed less than a year later by the consultant psychiatrist there was, according to his notes, 'quite strong evidence of an incipient psychosis'. He was prescribed chlorpromazine tablets, then referred to the psychiatric day hospital where he was found to be experiencing thought insertion, thought broadcasting, withdrawal, paranoid delusions, delusions of reference and auditory hallucinations. At this point he was prescribed a depot injection (fluphenazine). One year on, the psychiatrist recorded that he still found it difficult to make sense of Simon's experiences but regarded them as 'passivity phenomena, i.e. a schizophrenic first rank symptom' and it was suggested to Simon that he might have a 'schizophrenic disorder'. Simon also suffered from quite severe atopic eczema and asthma, and had a tendency to drink large amounts of alcohol. The following year he was admitted to the acute admissions ward and follow-up included continued support from the CPN and referral to the local social services day centre. It was at this point, four years after his initial presentation, that he was referred to me for BFT by his consultant.

At the time of our work together Simon was living in the family home. His mother, Denise, was 50 years old and had previously been treated for anxiety and depression (with antidepressants and an anxiety management group). His father, Vic, was 55 and headed the family business, although he was planning shortly to retire. Simon's younger brother, Steven, was 24 and lived in his own flat, although he visited the family regularly. He was currently working for the family business and the plan was he would take over the running of it when his father retired.

The idea of family intervention was introduced by Simon's CPN – a colleague of mine – who had also received training in BFT. We agreed to work together with the family and she introduced me to them. This was the first time we had worked with a family using this approach and we made this clear to them. We explained that the approach was well researched and had proven effectiveness, and that we were new to this way of working. For this reason we asked their permission to tape record the sessions so the recordings could be sent, confidentially, to our supervisor for evaluation and monitoring. They readily agreed and this may have helped the family to have confidence in the quality of the intervention. It also helped that they already had confidence in us as experienced CPNs.

Assessment

Following this first meeting (engagement), in the second session we carried out individual assessments with all four family members and at the following session assessed the family as a whole by examining their reported and observed problem-solving abilities. The individual assessments were done in one three-hour visit as, having started, the family preferred to get through this part of the process in one go. Much of this time was taken up allowing the parents to express their feelings about Simon's illness, which included confusion, irritation, sadness, denial and a range of emotions associated with grief and loss.

Formulation

This was the formulation we arrived at after the first three sessions:

> The family shares some common goals in the area of maintaining the family business with the burden of this shifting from Vic and Denise to Simon and Steven. Simon and Steven would like greater independence from their parents, while Vic and Denise equally would like to be more independent of Simon and Steven. Vic and Denise are struggling to cope with the negative effects of Simon's illness. Steven avoids this stress by spending time away and seems less aware of these difficulties. Simon finds his parents' frustration very stressful and an added burden to the illness itself. He is aware of a 'breakdown in communication' that he perceives as a lack of help. There is a general motivation and enthusiasm for change through BFT but the family's communication skills are generally poor, with the exception of Simon. Attempts at problem-solving are hampered by an inability to agree on a task and stick to it. Discussions are often circular and fuelled by anger. The family is able to generate ideas (even when they cannot keep the agreed problem in their sights) but tends to get side-tracked and is thus unable as a unit to evaluate options and plan a strategy. They need to clarify their respective roles (chair, secretary) and practise working in these roles.

What was striking about our formulation was that all the family members seemed to want similar things (greater independence from each other) and to have complementary goals (the parents wanting to relinquish responsibility for the family business, the two sons wanting to take on this responsibility). The early sessions were heated, characterised by raised voices and the family members constantly interrupting one another. This suggested that achieving the family's goals would be relatively easy if they could improve their communication skills. The parents found Simon's negative symptoms the most difficult aspect of the illness (rather than the positive symptoms). This is very much in keeping with the research on burden (Creer and Wing 1975; Vaughan 1977; Fadden *et al.* 1987). Steven had disengaged from the family somewhat and maintained this distance throughout the sessions, often arriving late and needing to leave early, or by eating, drinking or taking phone calls during the sessions. However, contrary to our initial predictions, he never completely disengaged and rarely missed a session.

Another striking feature of the formulation was the observation that it was Simon – the 'patient' – who seemed to have the best communication skills and the greatest insight into the family's communication problems. Family meetings without us present were to improve markedly once Vic (the self-elected chairman and generally the spokesperson for the family) abdicated this role and allowed Simon to chair the meetings. This seemed to encourage Vic to speak less and listen more actively.

Progress of sessions

After establishing the importance of a regular family meeting without us present (to practise skills and encourage independence from the therapists) we began a series of educational sessions in which we placed Simon as 'the expert on his own illness'. The sessions covered education about the illness, its symptoms and treatment, and the recognition of early warning signs of relapse. We also identified a need for an educational session on alcohol, how this related to the illness and its treatment, and the extent to which excessive use of alcohol was a problem, not just for Simon but for Steven too. In all, the educational sessions took six weeks, after which we used one session to review Vic and Denise's goals (to retire, move house and have a holiday without Simon) and another session to review Simon and Steven's goals (to take over the business and live in independent accommodation). It was gratifying that all four members of the family achieved all their goals by the end of our intervention.

After twelve sessions (which seemed quite slow progress from our point of view as therapists) we began communication skills training. The skills taught were expressing pleasant feelings, active listening, expressing negative feelings and making positive requests. Unfortunately, six months into the BFT, on Christmas Day, Simon was admitted to the acute admissions ward of the local psychiatric hospital under Section Three of the Mental Heath Act 1983. He had been experiencing symptoms of thought insertion and thought broadcasting. He also admitted to drinking about eight pints of beer every night and while on the ward was treated for alcohol withdrawal symptoms as well as for schizophrenic relapse.

In the New Year we wrote to the family and re-established the sessions, some of which took place at the hospital while Simon was still an in-patient. Notwithstanding the change of venue, all members of the family continued to make the effort to attend. Problem-solving became particularly necessary at this point and we introduced and taught the problem-solving technique at this stage. Communication skills training continued from January to October, and required considerable practice and revision. In November, Simon was again admitted to the ward, this time informally. His father had taken him to the hospital for assessment, having recognised the early warning signs of relapse and because he was also concerned about Simon's alcohol misuse. It was pleasing that, while the hospital admission was not prevented, intervention was early because of the family's awareness of the warning signs of relapse. It was also positive that this admission was informal rather than compulsory. Both admissions also seemed quite short for psychotic episodes, the first being for four weeks and the second only two weeks. The admitting psychiatrist recorded a diagnosis of 'schizophrenia, alcohol misuse'. Simon was experiencing visual hallucinations and, for the first time, admitted to experiencing auditory hallucinations.

Reflections

BFT is not only an evidence-based approach but one that seeks to promote reflective practice, which means both looking at what we, as therapists, did well and asking what we could have done differently that might have led to a better outcome. My own thoughts on this particular piece of family work were that, on the whole, it was successful and worthwhile but it felt labour-intensive and hard work at times. Working with families is not always easy and supervision is absolutely essential, not only to ensure fidelity to the approach and the development of skills but importantly also to protect therapists against disillusionment and demoralisation. It was somewhat disheartening to see Simon relapse and be admitted to hospital twice during the course of the BFT, given that it is known to be effective in preventing relapse and re-admission. This perhaps affected the credibility of BFT among our colleagues, particularly the consultant psychiatrist who had made the initial referral for BFT. It would have been better not to be embarrassed or demoralised by this perceived 'failure' of BFT but instead to look to the positive aspects: the unusually short admissions, Simon's speed of recovery and the change in his usual pattern of belated, compulsory admission to early, informal admission.

Overall, the intervention would probably have been more effective if we, as therapists, had not allowed the family – as they often did – to distract us from our planned session. It should not have been as long as six months before we introduced communication skills training. Nor should it have taken six months to work through this. Many sessions began with Vic or Denise saying: 'Can we just bring you up to date . . .' or 'There's just something we wanted to ask you before we start . . .' By the time we had discussed the particular concern there was little time left for the session we had planned. I did discuss this specific problem in BFT supervision and we subsequently decided to launch into the planned session at the beginning of each meeting and to deal with any current family concerns at the end. While this seemed a little unorthodox, we made better progress using this strategy.

Conclusions

Despite the setback of the second end-of-year admission, Simon's CPN and myself had already agreed to work towards disengaging from the family around this time. The family was communicating and problem-solving much more effectively. They had demonstrably greater knowledge and understanding of Simon's illness, and had been able to use their knowledge to seek help as soon as they recognised early warning signs of a relapse. They had also achieved all their goals. When Simon was discharged from his most recent admission we conducted a final educational session on dual diagnosis as it seemed clear alcohol misuse was a major factor in both his relapses and admissions. We followed the family up after a three-month interval (two years exactly from the start of our intervention) and their improvement had been maintained. The CPN continues to support Simon purely in her role as his CPN, rather than as family therapist, and the family continues to benefit from the knowledge and skills developed in the course of BFT.

Case study two: A case of things getting worse before they get better

Andrew

The identified patient Andrew (again, all names have been changed to protect the family's identity) is a 32-year-old man with a psychotic illness. He was first referred to psychiatric services when he was 22 years old, diagnosed as suffering from an acute schizophrenic psychosis. According to Andrew, he had been ill 'all his life really'. His mental condition, according to his initial assessment, had been slowly deteriorating since the age of 12 but he had only realised something was wrong when he became acutely psychotic. Four weeks prior to his admission, his behaviour had become increasingly abnormal and it was felt this was probably triggered off by the use of cannabis.

At initial assessment Andrew complained of auditory hallucinations, thought broadcasting/thought insertion, ideas of reference and passivity phenomena. In the past he had had delusions that he was Jesus and that aliens had landed on Earth, and he had paranoid ideas that everyone was against him.

Andrew's parents had divorced when he was 10, after his father had had a 'nervous breakdown'. His mother re-married when Andrew was 16. Andrew had had four brothers and one sister. His youngest brother died at the age of

16. Andrew had always been 'odd' and 'different'. When he was 15 it was considered he should see a child psychiatrist but this did not happen. He left school at 16, as his academic performance had begun to deteriorate. He did several unskilled jobs but did not hold on to them. A relationship with a girlfriend ended after three years, when she became pregnant by him. He had been in contact with the police for uninsured driving and stealing food. From the ages of 16 to 20 he smoked a lot of cannabis. He used to blame his 'weird thoughts' on the cannabis but discovered there was 'something wrong, which was not caused by the drugs'. He was admitted under Section Two of the Mental Health Act 1983 and was discharged to day hospital follow-up, on Fluphenazine, Procylidine and Prothiaden, his diagnosis having been changed to 'schizophrenia with an affective component'.

Andrew returned to living with his mother and step-father, and was reasonably well maintained on either oral anti-psychotics or a depot injection over the next nine years. The main destabilising factor seemed to be his experimentation with illicit drugs, including amphetamine. He was convicted of driving when intoxicated, resulting in a driving ban, and was fined for possession of cannabis. Around this time his sister abandoned her studies at university and returned home to live with Andrew and his mother, herself having presented with what appeared to be a psychotic illness.

The other household members

Andrew's mother (who shall here be called Norma) had been treated for depression in the past (with antidepressants). His sister ('Julie') was two years younger than Andrew. She had started a degree course at university but left after a psychotic episode. Andrew's step-father ('Mike') was also living in the household but Norma and Mike were separating at the time we started family interventions and are now divorced.

Engagement

I had been Andrew's CPN for about seven years prior to suggesting the 'new idea' of family intervention. It seemed very appropriate because, not only did Andrew have a diagnosis of schizophrenia (or schizo-affective illness) but Norma was clearly very stressed and communication in the house was often extremely negative. In addition, Julie (although not having been definitely diagnosed as having schizophrenia) had less well-defined mental health problems and seemed to experience psychotic and depressive phenomena intermittently. Julie was supported by a CPN colleague of mine. Although Julie's CPN had not undergone training in BFT, we agreed to co-work with the family since we both had a good relationship with different members of the family.

This was only the second family I had worked with using this approach and we made this clear to them. We explained that the approach was well researched and had proven effectiveness, and that we were new to this way of work. For this reason, we asked their permission to tape record the sessions so the recordings could be sent, confidentially, to our supervisor for evaluation and monitoring. Unfortunately, they declined to be tape recorded, a decision we had to respect.

Assessment

At the initial meeting with all four members of the household, Mike announced that he would not be taking part in future sessions as he would be moving out of the family home shortly. Neither myself nor Julie's CPN were fully aware that Mike's separation from Norma was so imminent.

We therefore agreed to work with the three remaining members of the household and carried out individual assessments with Andrew, Norma and Julie, and then assessed the family unit by examining their reported and observed problem-solving. The individual assessments were shared between myself and Julie's CPN. Time was taken to allow Norma, in particular, to express her feelings about Andrew's illness, Julie's illness and the death of her other son who had died of a physical illness. Norma spontaneously took the opportunity to discuss her dead son during the individual assessment. It seems Norma has never received any counselling or psychological support following this bereavement; although she had been treated with antidepressants. She was understandably anxious about Andrew's illness, his drug-taking and offending behaviour but felt more positive about Julie's problems, which she viewed more as a depressive rather than a schizophrenic illness.

Formulation

The following formulation was arrived at after the first three sessions (engagement, individual assessments and family assessment of problem-solving):

> Both Norma and Julie are enthusiastic about the offer of BFT. It is clear from the engagement sessions that Andrew is the most reluctant participant in the family intervention. He has expressed a fear that it could become just another opportunity for his mother and sister to criticise him. It is important to focus on goal-setting and communication skills, and to avoid focusing too much on those aspects of Andrew's behaviour which upset the rest of the family. Having said this, both Julie and Norma are keen to learn more about schizophrenia and especially the effect that Andrew's use of cannabis may have on his illness. The family's attempts at problem-solving were hampered by a lack of awareness about active listening skills (in particular their chosen seating arrangements meant that they were unable to have eye contact with one another), so communication skills training will be a priority. As regards individual

goals, Norma's revolve around further study or self-improvement and selling the house. The house sale is, of course, of concern to Andrew and Julie who live with her. Julie's goals involve returning to further education and getting fitter, while Andrew's centre on getting fitter and developing his interest in photography. There is scope for Andrew and Julie to work on their 'fitness goals' together, and for Julie and Norma to co-operate on their educational goals, but the question of the family home will probably need problem-solving once communication skills have been improved.

What was striking about our formulation was that some of the family members' goals were similar (further education, improved fitness) but others could potentially cause great conflict (e.g. Norma's desire to sell the house while Julie and Andrew were living there). The early sessions were characterised by Andrew's sporadic attendance. Often Norma and Julie would start the session attentively but would be anxious and annoyed at Andrew's lateness or non-attendance. We decided we would proceed with sessions regardless but that we would all remind Andrew in between sessions of the subsequent appointment times. Family meetings without the therapists did take place but, again, it was usually the two women who cajoled Andrew into joining them for these. Julie, in particular, seemed to enjoy the role of secretary and would present minutes from family meetings at some of our sessions. Andrew, however, seemed to experience this as further evidence of the women controlling his life.

Progress of sessions

We began with a series of educational sessions in which we encouraged Andrew and Julie to 'compare notes' about their experience of mental health problems. We tried to emphasise that they were 'the experts on their own illnesses'. Unfortunately, this sometimes descended into a comparison of who gets which symptoms and what might be inferred from this in terms of diagnosis. Julie seemed keen to 'find out' if she had schizophrenia or not, while Andrew seemed convinced that he had been correctly diagnosed and felt (like Norma) that Julie's illness was more likely to be depression (of which all three have had experience). In response to pressure from Norma and Julie, we included some education on cannabis and its relationship to mental health. We experienced some difficulty obtaining reliable information on this subject and approached the community drugs team to see if they could offer some input. Unfortunately, this was not forthcoming.

Increasingly, Andrew's attendance deteriorated and the other family members expressed concern that he was not taking his medication and was showing early signs of relapse. They also suspected he was using increasing amounts of illicit drugs. We had discussed early warning signs of relapse but Andrew seemed unco-operative about this at this stage.

We began communication skills training (the skills taught being expressing pleasant feelings, active listening, expressing negative feelings and making positive requests). At the sessions Andrew attended, he appeared to have a good understanding of the communication skills and found it helpful to express his feelings to his mother in particular. Unfortunately, it appeared as if Andrew was beginning to relapse and he gradually disengaged from the family interventions. Because of the good relationship we had developed with the family as a result of BFT, we were able to discuss (in Andrew's absence) how best to help him. Although he was expressing paranoid ideas about his family, he was also surprisingly amenable to my visits (partly because of my long-standing relationship with Andrew as his CPN but also, perhaps, because of the greater investment of time I had made through the BFT).

Soon after this, I learnt that Andrew had become aggressive towards his family and had then decided to go to Amsterdam for a few days on his own. On his return, I was called to see him at the house by Julie who told me Norma had moved out temporarily. Andrew told me guardedly about his visit to Amsterdam and how deeply affected he had been by seeing the effects of drugs on various 'down-and-outs' on the streets. He had decided to return home but was clearly in a fragile mental state, having had no medication for some time. I persuaded him to come into hospital for an informal admission, so that we could help him recover from his drug abuse and to give the family a break. He agreed to this and, after a few days as an in-patient, with his antipsychotic medication reinstated, he appeared much better.

A few weeks later, Andrew stopped to chat with me in the hospital reception area and told me how he had been using the communication skills to deal with difficult fellow patients on the ward. He had decided that he wanted to go to a mental health rehabilitation hostel rather than return to the family home. This was arranged upon discharge and Andrew managed to remain on medication and free of illicit drugs while living in the hostel. He also asked me to review his early warning signs of relapse with him and to share this with his key worker at the hostel. Furthermore, Andrew found a new girl-friend in the form of a fellow resident and they have now both moved out into shared accommodation and are planning to marry soon.

Andrew has achieved his goal of becoming physically fitter, having stopped the use of illicit drugs and having taken up cycling, body building and Tai Kwan Do. He is managing to avoid the weight gain associated with his medication through vigorous regular exercise.

Reflections

According to Andrew, he had been ill 'all his life really'. His mental condition, according to his initial assessment, had been slowly deteriorating since the age of 12 but he had only realised something was wrong when he became acutely psychotic. This is surely a powerful argument for early intervention in psychosis. It is interesting to note that referral to a child psychiatrist was suggested ten years prior to Andrew's first admission but that this did not occur. Had Andrew received help from child and adolescent services, or even early intervention services in adulthood, his deterioration resulting in a compulsory admission and protracted recovery may have been averted.

As therapists we were rather wrong-footed when, at the engagement stage, Mike announced he was moving out of the family home. Had we nurtured closer relationships with the other family members prior to suggesting BFT, we might have been more aware that Norma and Mike's relationship was ending and this could have been taken into account at the onset of BFT. The lesson to be learnt here seems to be that forging good, communicative relationships with families and carers should not wait till, or depend upon, the offer of structured family intervention.

There were a number of questions raised by Andrew's drug use and how this was approached within the context of BFT. The inclusion of some education on cannabis and its relationship to mental health was in response to pressure from Norma and Julie, who seemed to hope that it might help Andrew to 'see sense', as it were. This may, inadvertently, have increased Andrew's feeling that the BFT was a vehicle for his mother and sister to criticise and pressurise him into changing his behaviour. On a practical level, the fact that we experienced some difficulty obtaining reliable information on the effects of cannabis on mental health highlights the need for better liaison between community drugs workers and generic mental health services. There is growing awareness of dual diagnosis (e.g. schizophrenia accompanied by drug or alcohol misuse – as was the case in both the case studies here). Despite this, it is a disappointing but common observation that generic mental health workers do not feel confident in managing substance misuse, while substance misuse specialists do not feel confident in managing mental illness. This gap needs to be addressed by training and organisational structures.

It could be argued that BFT exacerbated a crisis in Andrew that resulted in his relapse and readmission. This, of course, is ironic given that these are two factors known to be positively affected by BFT. Moreover, the intervention did not seem, in the short term, to have improved compliance with medication. However, if a long-term view is taken, it could be said that the intervention has resulted in greater compliance, better management of the illness, reduced stress for the other family members, improved overall health and greater independence for Andrew. Although achieved by rather a tortuous route, it is hard to know whether these outcomes could have been achieved without relapse, re-admission and rehabilitation. Perhaps the BFT precipitated the crisis that was needed to bring about change.

Conclusions

It being the second family with whom I had used this approach, my expectations were different. I was able to take a more positive view of the outcomes, even if these were not the ones predicted. Non-compliance, relapse and re-admission are not necessarily signs of failure in the approach, so long as they result in long-term improved compliance and reduced frequency of relapse and re-admission. That Andrew, even when quite unwell, was able to use knowledge and skills developed through BFT to deal assertively with his situation is extremely encouraging. That he and other family members appear to be leading more independent, healthy and satisfying lives is all that we – as mental health workers – could ask.

References

2 No such thing as society – sociological aspects of community psychiatric nursing

Reflection

Clarke, L. (1999). *Challenging Ideas in Psychiatric Nursing*. Routledge, London.

'Community' and 'neighbourhood' – how concepts shape the provision of care

Abercrombie, N., Hill, S. and Turner, B. S. (1988). *Penguin Dictionary of Sociology*. Penguin, Harmondsworth.

Cobb, A. (1990). News item in 'Mind's Eye', *Open Mind*, 45, June/July: 9.

Cumberlege, J. and the Community Nursing Review (1986). *Neighbourhood Nursing – A Focus for Care*. (Report of the Community Nursing Review Team.) HMSO, London.

Dennis, N. (1968). 'The popularity of the neighbourhood community ideas', in Pahl, R. (ed.) *Readings in Urban Sociology*. Pergamon Press, London.

MacIver, R. M. and Page, C. H. (1961). *Society: An introductory analysis*. Macmillan, London.

Piaget, J. (1929). *The Child's Conception of the World*. Routledge & Kegan Paul, London.

Toennies, F. (1955). *Community and Association*. (Originally published 1887.) Routledge & Kegan Paul, London.

Townsend, S. (1989). *Mr Bevan's Dream*. Counterblasts series. Chatto & Windus, London.

Webber, M. (1979). Excerpt from 'The urban place and the non-place urban realm', in Worsley, P. (ed.), *Modern Sociology – Introductory Readings*. Penguin, Harmondsworth.

Wirth, L. (1979). Excerpt from 'The scope and problems of the community', in Worsley, P. (ed.), *Modern Sociology – Introductory Readings*. Penguin, Harmondsworth.

Unemployment links with mental health

Chapman, C. (1982). *Sociology for Nurses*. Baillière Tindall, London.

Rees, L. (1982). *A Short Textbook of Psychiatry*, 3rd edition. Hodder & Stoughton, London.

Get the bucket and mop, nurse

Keillor, G. (1986). *Lake Wobegon Days.* Faber & Faber, London.
United Kingdom Central Council (UKCC) (1992). *Register*, 11, Oct.

3 A day in the life – the role of the Community Psychiatric Nurse

Reflection

Benner, P. and Wrubel, J. (1989). *The Primacy of Caring: Stress and coping in health and illness.* Addison-Wesley Publishing Company, California.
Johnstone, L. (2000). *Users and Abusers of Psychiatry: A critical look at psychiatric practice*, 2nd edition. Routledge, London.

The role of community mental health workers

Clare, A. and Corney, R. (eds) (1982). *Social Work and Primary Health Care.* Academic Press, London.
Department of Health and Social Security (1968). *Report of the Committee on Local Authority and Allied Personal Services.* HMSO, London.
English National Boards for Nursing, Midwifery and Health Visiting (ENB) (1987). *Syllabus of Training 1982 for the Professional Register Part Three.* ENB, London.
Griffith, J. and Mangen, S. (1980). Community psychiatric nursing – a literature review. *International Journal of Nursing Studies*, 17: 197–210.
Horder, J. (1986). 'Professional team roles', in Shepherd, M., Wilkinson, G. and Williams, P. (eds), *Mental Illness in Primary Care Settings.* Tavistock, London.
Huxley, P. (1991). 'Social work', in Bennett, D. and Freeman, H. (eds), *Community Psychiatry.* Churchill Livingstone, Edinburgh.
Jefferys, M. (1986). 'Professional team roles', in Shepherd, M., Wilkinson, G. and Williams, P. (eds), *Mental Illness in Primary Care Settings.* Tavistock, London.
May, A. and Moore, S. (1963). The mental nurse in the community. *The Lancet*, 1: 213–214.
Morrall, P. (1989). The professionalisation of community psychiatric nursing. *Community Psychiatric Nursing Journal*, 9 (4): 14–22.
Rawlinson, J. and Brown, A. (1991). 'Community psychiatric nursing in Britain', in Bennett, D. and Freeman, H. (eds), *Community Psychiatry.* Churchill Livingstone, Edinburgh.
Skidmore, D. and Friend, W. (1984). Community psychiatric nursing. *Community Outlook*, 80: 19.
Sladden, S. (1979). *Psychiatric Nursing in the Community.* Churchill Livingstone, Edinburgh.
White, E. (1990). *Community Psychiatric Nursing: The 1990 Survey.* Community Psychiatric Nurses Association, Nuneaton.
Wooff, K. *et al.* (1988). The practice of community psychiatric nursing and mental health social work in Salford. Some implications for community care. *British Journal of Psychiatry*, 152: 783–792.
Wooff, K. and Goldberg, D. (1988). Further observations on the practice of

community care in Salford. Differences between community psychiatric nurses and mental health social workers. *British Journal of Psychiatry*, 153: 30–37.

4 Learning in lay-bys – teaching and assessing

Reflection

Bowles, N. (1995). Story telling: a search for meaning within nursing practice. *Nurse Education Today*, 15: 365–369.
Sacks, O. (1986). *The Man Who Mistook His Wife for a Hat.* Picador, London.

Teaching and learning in lay-bys – applying reflective practice to teaching in the community

Benner, P. (1984). *From Novice to Expert: Power and excellence in clinical nursing.* Jossey-Bass, Menlo Park, California.
Bowles, N. (1995). Story telling: a search for meaning within nursing practice. *Nurse Education Today*, 15: 365–369.
Burnard, P. (1989). Experiential learning and andragogy – negotiated learning in nurse education: a critical appraisal. *Nurse Education Today*, 9: 300–306.
Burrows, D. E. (1995). The nurse teacher's role in the promotion of reflective practice. *Nurse Education Today*, 15: 346–350.
English and Welsh National Boards for Nursing, Midwifery and Health Visiting (1982). *Syllabus of Training: Part 3 (Registered Mental Nurse).* ENB, Milton Keynes.
Gournay, K. (1995). Training and education in mental health nursing. *Mental Health Nursing*, 15 (6): 12–14.
Heron, J. (1986). *Six Category Intervention Analysis.* Human Potential Research Project, University of Surrey, Guildford.
Holt, J. (1969). *How Children Fail.* Pelican Books (Penguin), Harmondsworth.
Merchant, J. (1989). The challenge of experiential methods in nursing education. *Nurse Education Today*, 9: 307–313.
Milligan, F. (1995). In defence of andragogy. *Nurse Education Today*, 15: 22–27.
United Kingdom Central Council (UKCC) (1986). *Project 2000: A new preparation for practice.* UKCC, London.

Reflection

Dickens, C. (1854, published in Penguin 1969). *Hard Times.* Penguin, Harmondsworth.
Milligan, F. (1995). In defence of andragogy. *Nurse Education Today*, 15: 22–27.

Taking a humanistic approach to assessment – the assessment of nursing competence in the community

Ashworth, P. and Morrison, P. (1991). Problems of competence-based nurse education. *Nurse Education Today*, 11: 256–260.
Bowles, N. (1995). Story telling: a search for meaning within nursing practice. *Nurse Education Today*, 15: 365–369.

Boydell, T. (1976). *Experiential Learning*. Manchester Monographs. Manchester.

Burnard, P. (1989). Experiential learning and andragogy – negotiated learning in nurse education: a critical appraisal. *Nurse Education Today*, 9: 300–306.

Burnard, P. (1994). *Counselling Skills for Health Professionals*, 2nd edition. Chapman & Hall, London.

Cook, S. H. (1991). Mind the theory/practice gap in nursing. *Journal of Advanced Nursing*, 18: 621–626.

English and Welsh National Boards for Nursing, Midwifery and Health Visiting (1982). *Syllabus of Training: Part 3 (Registered Mental Nurse)*. ENB, Milton Keynes.

English National Board (ENB) (1987). *Managing Change in Nursing Education. Pack 1*. ENB, Milton Keynes.

English National Board (ENB) (1988). *Institutional and Course Approval/Reapproval Process: Information required, criteria and guidelines*. Circular 1988/39/APS. ENB, London.

Everett, A. (1995). The educational role of the community mental health nurse. *Mental Health Nursing*, 15 (5): 8–10.

Merchant, J. (1989). The challenge of experiential methods in nursing education. *Nurse Education Today*, 9: 307–313.

Milligan, F. (1995). In defence of andragogy. *Nurse Education Today*, 15: 22–27.

Phillips, T., Bedford, H., Robinson, J. and Schostak, J. (1994). *Education, Dialogue and Assessment: Creating partnership for improving practice*. ENB, London.

Reader's Digest (1987). *Universal Dictionary*. Reader's Digest Association Limited, London.

Sarosi, G. M. and O'Connor, P. (1993). The microstory pathway of executive nursing rounds: tales of living caring. *Nursing Administration Quarterly*, 17 (2): 30–37.

United Kingdom Central Council (UKCC) (1986). *Project 2000: A new preparation for practice*. UKCC, London.

Young, A. (1994). *Law and Professional Conduct in Nursing*, 2nd edition. Scutari Press, Harrow.

5 Risky business – risk-taking and safe practice

Reflection

Bagley, H. (1996). *Learning Materials in Mental Health*. St Martin's Press, New York.

Risk-taking: a nurse's duty

Carson, D. (1990). 'Taking risks with patients – your assessment strategy', in *The Staff Nurse's Survival Guide*. Austin Cornish, London.

Oxford University Press (OUP) (1982). *Concise Oxford Dictionary*. OUP, Oxford.

Reader's Digest (1987). *Universal Dictionary*. Reader's Digest Association Limited, London.

United Kingdom Central Council (UKCC) (1984). *Code of Professional Conduct for the Nurse, Midwife and Health Visitor*, 2nd edition. UKCC, London.

United Kingdom Central Council (UKCC) (1989). *Exercising Accountability*. UKCC, London.

Some thoughts on clinical supervision

Farrington, A. (1998). Clinical supervision: issues for mental health nursing. *Mental Health Nursing*, 18 (1): 19–21.

6 If you're happy and you know it – promoting positive mental health

Reflection

Department of Health (2000). *A National Service Framework for Mental Health.* DoH, London. http: //www.doh.gov.uk/pub/docs/doh/mhmain/pdf.
Keillor, G. (1986). *Lake Wobegon Days.* Faber & Faber, London.

7 Totally atypical taste – coming to terms with newer treatments

Reflection

O'Brien, M. and Houston, G. (2000). *Integrative Therapy: A practitioner's guide.* Sage Publications, London.

Representational systems in counselling

Bandler, R. and Grinder, J. (1979). *Frogs Into Princes.* Real People Press, New York.
Geldard, D. (1989). *Basic Personal Counselling.* Prentice-Hall, Sydney.
O'Connor, J. and Seymour, J. (1990). *Introducing Neuro-Linguistic Programming.* Crucible, London.
Wilson, H. S. and Kneisl, C. R. (1988). *Psychiatric Nursing.* Addison-Wesley, Menlo Park, California.

Reflection

Healy, D. (1999). *The Antidepressant Era.* Harvard University Press, Cambridge, Massachusetts.
James, O. (1998). *Britain on the Couch: Why we're unhappier than we were in the 1950s – despite being richer.* Century Random House, London.

Reflection

Clarke, L. (1999). *Challenging Ideas in Psychiatric Nursing.* Routledge, London.
Sladden, S. (1979). *Psychiatric Nursing in the Community.* Churchill Livingstone, Edinburgh.

Schizophrenia and atypical antipsychotics

Colonna, L., Saleem, P., Dondey-Nouvel, L., Rein, W. and the Amisulpride Study Group (2000). Long-term safety and efficacy of amisulpride in subchronic or chronic schizophrenia. *International Clinical Psychopharmacology*, 15: 13–22.

Dratcu, L. (2000). Antipsychotic formulations. *Community Mental Health*, 2 (4): 10–14.
Gournay, K. and Gray, R. (1998). The role of new drugs in the treatment of schizo-phrenia. *Mental Health Nursing*, 18 (2): 21–24.
Mari, J. J., Adams, C. E. and Streiner, D. (1997). 'Family interventions for schizo-phrenia', in Adams, C. E., De Jesus Mari, J. and White, P. (eds), *Schizophrenia Module of the Cochrane Database of Systematic Reviews*. Update Software/The Cochrane Collaboration (updated quarterly), Oxford.

8 Reintegration through creativity

Reflection

Goddard, J. (1996). *Mixed Feelings: Littlemore Hospital – an oral history project*. Oxfordshire County Council, Oxford.
Morris, R. (1998). *Shelton Past and Present*. Shropshire's Community and Mental Health Services NHS Trust, Shrewsbury.

Creative arts as therapy

Yalom, I. D. (1986). *The Theory and Practice of Group Psychotherapy*. Basic Books, New York.

Sounds good – establishing therapeutic music groups in community mental health settings

Alvin, J. (1975). *Music Therapy*. Hutchinson, London.
Benenzon, R.O. (1981). *Music Therapy Manual*. Charles C. Thomas, Springfield, Illinois.
Bunt, L. (1994). *Music Therapy – An art beyond words*. Routledge, London.

9 True colours – working with primary care

Managing depression in primary care – the role of the practice nurse

Blenkiron, P. (1998). The management of depression in primary care: a summary of evidence-based guidelines. *Psychiatric Care*, 5 (5):172–177.
Cook, R. (1999). Setting standards for quality healthcare. *Practice Nurse*, 17: 590–595.
Nolan, P., Dunn, L. and Badger, F. (1998). Getting to know you. *Nursing Times*, 94 (39): 34–36.
Paykel, E. S. and Priest, R. G. (1992). Recognition and management of depression in general practice: Consensus statement. *British Medical Journal*, 305: 1198–1202.
Royal College of General Practitioners (RCGP) (1993). *Shared Care of Patients with Mental Health Problems*. (Occasional paper no. 60.) RCGP, London.

Putting innovation on the map

Borrow, G. (1977, first published 1862). *Wild Wales – its people, language and scenery*. Collins, Glasgow.

Department of Health (1992). *The Health of the Nation: A strategy for health in England*. HMSO, London.

10 We are family – family interventions

Family therapy – exploring the role of the CPN

Carr, P. J., Butterworth, C. A. and Hodges, B. E. (1980). *Community Psychiatric Nursing*. Churchill Livingstone, Edinburgh.

Clayton, G. (1989). Family therapy – theory meets practice. *Community Care*, 30 March.

Cooper, G. (1987). Mental health nursing: the family way. *Nursing Times*, 83 (18), May 6–12.

McDonald, N. (1987). Psychiatric skills: ask the family. *Nursing Times*, 83 (3), Jan. 21–27.

McMahon, B. (1990). Helping families towards open communication. *Professional Nurse*, Apr.

Minuchin, S. (1974). *Families and Family Therapy*. Harvard University Press, Cambridge, Massachusetts; London.

Pollock, L. (1989). *Community Psychiatric Nursing: Myth and reality*. Royal College of Nursing (RCN) Research series, Scutari Press, Harrow.

Sheehy, B. (1990). Three years on: CPN-run family therapy clinic. *Community Psychiatric Nursing Journal*, 10 (3), June.

Simmons, S. and Brooker, C. (1986). *Community Psychiatric Nursing: A social perspective*. Heinemann, London.

Walrond-Skinner, S. (1976). *Family Therapy*. Routledge & Kegan Paul, London.

The case for using family interventions in the management of schizophrenia

Anderson, C. M., Griffin, S. and Rossi, A. (1986). A comparative study of the impact of education vs process groups for families with affective disorders. *Fam Process*, 25: 185–205.

Backer, T. E., Liberman, R. P. and Kuehnel, T. G. (1986). Dissemination and adoption of innovative psychosocial interventions. *J. Consulting Clin Psychol*, 54: 111–118.

Brennan, G. and Gamble, C. (1997). Schizophrenia family work and clinical practice. *Mental Health Nurs*, 17 (4): 12–15.

Brown, G. W., Birley, J. L. T. and Wing, J. K. (1972). Influence of family life on the course of schizophrenic disorder. *Br. J. Psychiatry*, 121: 241–258.

Clarkin, J. F., Glick, I. D. and Haas, G. L. (1990). A randomised clinical trial of inpatient family intervention v. results for affective disorders. *J. Affective Dis*, 18: 17–28.

Droogan, J. and Brannigan, K. (1997). A review of psychosocial family interventions for schizophrenia. *Nursing Times*, 93 (26): 46–47.

Fadden, G. (1997). Implementation of family interventions in routine clinical practice following staff training programmes: a major cause for concern. *J. Mental Health*, 6: 599–612.

Fadden, G. (1998). Research update: psychoeducational family interventions. *Journal of Family Therapy*, 20 (3): 293–309.

Falloon, I. (1998). 'Cognitive–behavioural interventions for patients with functional psychoses and their caregivers: an annotated bibliography', in *World Schizophrenia Fellowship Strategy Document: Families as Partners in Care*. World Schizophrenia Fellowship, Toronto.

Falloon, I., Mueser, K. and Gingerich, S. (1996). *Behavioural Family Therapy – A workbook*, 2nd edition. Buckingham Mental Health Service, Buckingham: Busiprint Ltd.

Furlong, M. and Leggatt, M. (1996). Reconciling the patient's right to confidentiality and the family's need to know. *Aus NZ J Psychiatry*, 30: 614–622.

Gillam, T. (1994). CPN'd of the line? *Nursing Standard*, 8 (18): 45–46.

Gillam, T. (1998). Too close for comfort? *Nursing Times*, 94 (39): 35.

Glick, I. D., Burti, L. and Okonogi, K. (1994). Effectiveness in psychiatric care, III. Psychoeducation and outcome for patients with major affective disorder and their families. *Br J Psychiatry*, 164: 104–106.

Goldstein, M. J. and Miklowitz, D. J. (1994). Family intervention for persons with bipolar disorder. *New Directions Mental Health Services*, 62: 23–35.

Kavanagh, D. J., Tennant, C. and Rosen, A. (1988). *Prevention of Relapse in Schizophrenia*. Research and Development Grant, Commonwealth Department of Community Services and Health.

Kottgen, C., Sonnichsen, I. and Mollenhauer, K. (1984). Group therapy with families of schizophrenia patients: results of the Hamburg Camberwell Family Interview study III. *Int J Fam Psych*, 5: 83–94.

Leff, J., Kuipers, L. and Berkowitz, R. (1982). A controlled trial of social intervention in the families of schizophrenic patients. *Br J Psychiatry*, 141: 121–134.

Mari, J. J., Adams, C. E. and Streiner, D. (1997). 'Family interventions for schizophrenia', in Adams, C. E., De Jesus Mari, J. and White, P. (eds), *Schizophrenia Module of the Cochrane Database of Systematic Reviews*. Update Software/The Cochrane Collaboration, Oxford.

McCreadie, R. G., Phillips, K. and Harvey, J. A. (1991). The Nithsdale Schizophrenia Surveys VIII. Do relatives want family intervention – and does it help? *Br J Psychiatry*, 158: 110–113.

McFarlane, W. R. (1994). Multiple family groups and psychoeducation in the treatment of schizophrenia. *New Directions Mental Health Services*, 62: 13–23.

Szmukler, G. I. and Bloch, S. (1997). Family involvement in the care of people with psychoses: an ethical argument. *Br J Psychiatry*, 171: 401–405.

Vaughan, K., Doyle, M. and Mcconahy, N. (1992). The Sydney Intervention Trial: a controlled trial of relatives' counselling to reduce schizophrenia relapse. *Soc Psychiatry Psychiatr Epidemiol*, 27: 16–21.

Two case studies of psychoeducational family interventions

Creer, C. and Wing, J. (1975). Living with a schizophrenic patient. *British Journal of Hospital Medicine*, 14: 73–82.

Fadden, G., Bebbington, P. and Kuipers, L. (1987). The burden of care: the impact of functional psychiatric illness on the patient's family. *British Journal of Psychiatry*, 150: 285–292.

Vaughan, C. E. (1977). 'Patterns of interactions in families of schizophrenics', in Katschnig, H., *Schizophrenia: The other side*. Urban & Schwarzenberg, Vienna.

Index

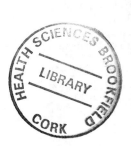